Homebirth
in the
Hospital

HOMEBIRTH IN THE HOSPITAL

Integrating Natural Childbirth with Modern Medicine

STACEY MARIE KERR MD

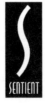

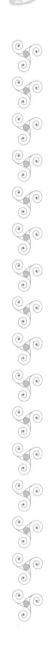

A paperback original

Cover design by Kim Johansen, Black Dog Design
Book design by Elizabeth Lahey, Envisible Graphics

Library of Congress Cataloging-in-Publication Data

Kerr, Stacey Marie, 1949-
   Homebirth in the hospital : integrating natural childbirth with modern medicine / by Stacey Marie Kerr.
      p. cm.
   ISBN 978-1-59181-077-3
   1. Natural childbirth. 2. Childbirth. 3. Integrative medicine. I. Title.
   RG661.K48 2008
   618.4—dc22

                              2008003532

Printed in the United States of America

10 9 8 7 6 5 4 3 2 1

SENTIENT PUBLICATIONS
A Limited Liability Company
1113 Spruce Street
Boulder, CO 80302
www.sentientpublications.com

This book is dedicated to my teachers, both midwives and MDs, and to the nurses at Santa Rosa Community Hospital—for the support they have provided, for the faith they have in my style and skills, and for making it possible to promise care that fosters empowerment, not fear.

CONTENTS

CONTENTS

CONTENTS

INTRODUCTION

I thought about Kathryn as I drove out River Road in the dark, hunched over my steering wheel and peering out the windshield past wipers that were vainly trying to clear torrential rain. She was thirty-nine years old, with a very precocious daughter. She had a history of drug abuse—alcohol, cigarettes, and various illegal substances—but all of these were in her distant past. Her daughter Maggie had been born in the hospital seven years ago after an induced labor at forty-two weeks—four and a half pounds quickly pushed out after an episiotomy (a surgical incision through the perineum to enlarge the vagina). This time Kathryn had decided to birth at home; her labor tonight had been induced with castor oil, and I knew she had been working hard all day. The midwives hadn't called me until dusk was closing in on the Russian River Valley, so I fully expected to miss the delivery as I drove up and down the Bohemian Highway, lost in the rain and the dark.

When I finally found the small cottage tucked under the redwoods, I parked next to the road and made my way inside. The door opened to a bright and steamy kitchen where Dan, Kathryn's brother, and Suzette, one of the midwives, were making a spaghetti dinner for the group. The air in the cottage was close after the freshness of the cold rain outside. The woodstove was cranking out heat and I was assaulted by the strong aromas of wood smoke, spaghetti sauce, and the yeasty scent of a woman long in labor. I knew immediately that I was not too late. Clearly, this was a group that had been working together all day and they were glad for my fresh face and energy.

For me, this journey through the rain was part of my residency training as a family practice physician. Midway through my training, I had the opportunity to take a month-long elective in homebirth. With the support of my advisors, I had made agreements with two local midwives to attend births with them. I was not here to provide medical backup; I was only to be an observer on the scene. These midwives were well-known, well-respected certified nurse-midwives with hospital privileges. My medical teachers were reassured that I would be in good hands, and I was ecstatic about being allowed to attend births with no beeping machines to dilute the experience. And so it was that I found myself in Kathryn's kitchen, bringing in fresh air and a new perspective. I was attending this homebirth because I knew I wanted to revisit the midwife way of birthing after months of training at hospital births. What I didn't know was that this was a birth that would help shape my future style of practice.

Declining a plate of spaghetti, I made my way back to the bedroom to find that Kathryn had just begun to push. Her sister-in-law and little Maggie, Kathryn's daughter, were helping her by providing cool washcloths for her face and sips of juice to keep her strength up. Carolyn, the other midwife, smiled up at me from where she sat in the corner, letting the family take care of Kathryn for the time being.

After saying hello to the birthing party, I settled down next to Carolyn and she quietly brought me up to date. "I just spent some time working a stubborn anterior lip out of the way. It's staying up behind the baby's head now so it's only a matter of time. She's a good pusher."

I saw Kathryn was pushing in earnest but it didn't look like this baby was going to slither right out like Maggie had. This one was going to take some work. So we waited.

Kathryn's brother Dan came in to support the pushing efforts. I had never seen such a watermelon-like belly; it was sticking straight out, firm, round, and darkly veined. Huge. I could not stop staring at that belly and wondering how long it would take Kathryn to get this baby out. The midwives and I watched and assisted for the next two hours while Kathryn pushed valiantly from many different positions. First she pushed on her hands and knees. Then, with Dan supporting her weight from behind, she squatted—a squat made difficult by the swelling in her legs and feet. Her belly tightened and enlarged with each contraction until I thought she would burst. We were monitoring the baby's heartbeat with a portable Doppler every fifteen minutes or so. After a while the baby started showing some distress during the contractions. We heard some temporary heart-rate decelerations, so for about twenty minutes we monitored each contraction. We moved Kathryn around, trying to help the baby. First we had her lie on her left side, then her right. After a bit of this maneuvering, and a few more contractions, the baby recovered and never again showed any signs of distress. I couldn't help but notice the midwife's response to the baby's distress. It was so different than what I saw back at the hospital. She was watchful and concerned but gave the baby time to recover after each contraction without intervening from a place of panic or fear. She was not overreacting, and I felt my own tension ease as I watched her work.

Kathryn leaned back on Dan's chest, sitting up in bed to push. The sheets were damp. The air in the cabin was close and stale. I opened the door to the rain outside, letting in some fresh air to mix with the warmth of the fire. Kathryn waddled to the toilet, sat on it, and pushed for half an hour. Then she worked on her hands and knees next to the bathtub. Her sister crouched next to her, lightly resting her hand on Kathryn's back in between contractions. Kathryn was looking every bit her thirty-nine years and then some. She lumbered up off the bathroom floor and made her way back into the bedroom. At one point she stood up with Dan's support during a contraction, and as she pushed the two midwives pushed hard and inward on her hips to flare the pelvic outlet (the opening at the lower border of the pelvis). I had never seen this done before. Although it looked very primitive, it also looked like something that might help Kathryn get this baby out. I crouched in front of her and peered at her vagina, looking for the first glimpse of the baby's head. Nothing. Finally she came back to the squatting stool.

She was making very slow progress, and I was starting to get a little anxious. The baby's head was still not moving past the bones of Kathryn's pelvis. What would the midwives do now? I wondered if we should consider doing something more aggressive to help Kathryn before she ran out of energy and simply gave up. Wasn't this becoming a high-risk situation?

It was then that I noticed Carolyn in the kitchen, talking on the phone. Grabbing a piece of garlic bread off the counter, I moved closer to hear what she was saying and listened to her consult with her obstetrical backup in town. She was reporting on the slow progress, checking in, and letting the doctor know that we were still working on getting this baby out. She didn't sound too worried, but then Carolyn never does let herself sound worried. She's known for keeping calm in almost any situation; she is a seasoned midwife.

Kathryn said later that when she saw her midwife on the phone, she assumed they were talking about taking her to the hospital. What she did not realize was that the rainstorm had temporarily washed out the roads by the river, and a trip to town would have been very difficult if not impossible. Fortunately, this was the moment when Kathryn decided to have the baby. She didn't say anything and her outward behavior didn't change, but she felt a new and strong determination. She knew she needed to get this baby out and she needed to do it soon.

We wanted her to stand up and push, but she was physically exhausted. Dan tried to support her. He stood behind her and gripped her under her arms, giving her his full weight to lean against. She was protesting weakly, "No! I can't! Really! I need to…" when a contraction came and before she could finish protesting she was forced to push while standing up. Kneeling in front of her, I looked up at Dan, wondering if he had the strength to hold her. He had a look of determination and concentration that I didn't want to challenge; his legs were planted firmly against his sister's thighs. I crouched down lower to watch her vagina and caught my breath when I realized I was seeing my first view of her baby's head, the wet dark hair moving down well past the pubic bone. This is what we had been waiting for! "Carolyn! Now!" I said as I moved out of the way quickly, letting her in so that she could catch the baby.

I couldn't believe how fast it happened once things finally started moving. Kathryn sank into a squat in spite of her fat ankles. With nothing now to stop it, the baby kept coming down and out. The cord was wrapped four times around his neck but Carolyn worked quickly to untangle it, slipping the loops over the baby's head and suctioning his nose. Then all nine pounds, four ounces were delivered, sliding into Carolyn's waiting hands in one smooth move. Little Maggie stared over my shoulder, watching in awe as the midwife guided her brother out inch by inch. Finally, Kathryn sat back on a stool and held her wet warm baby boy to her breasts. She had done it, and her look of exhausted sweaty satisfaction was one I will never forget.

Ten minutes later, with Kathryn still squatting on the stool, the placenta delivered easily along with about a cup and a half of dark blood. She and

Carolyn looked at it together, this organ that had supported her son for nine months. They touched the translucent membranes, stretching the rent through which the birth had moved, and they explored the rough surface that had been bonded to her uterus and was now no longer needed. The long cord lay flaccid among the membranes.

Now we were able to help Kathryn move to the bed where she could be more comfortable, and it was during this move that I saw some ragged tearing on her perineum. I couldn't be sure, but it looked like we had some fancy sewing to do before we were done. I looked over at Carolyn, catching her eye with a look of cautious alarm. She smiled at me in a reassuring way and commented out loud, "Looks good, Kathryn. Not much bleeding right now at all. Let me check your bottom and then we'll let you be." Her comments were as much for me as they were for Kathryn, although I don't think Kathryn was worried about anything right then; she was completely immersed in the sight, smell, and reality of her newborn son. Carolyn took a minute to look at Kathryn's perineum, feeling it with her hands and using a flashlight to see. Her expression remained calm, so I naively figured it must not have been as bad as I thought. We tucked Kathryn into bed with her baby and moved into the kitchen to give this new little family some time together to bond.

Standing around the remains of a half-eaten spaghetti dinner, the two midwives and I munched on cold garlic bread while we discussed the birth. Out of sight and speaking softly so she wouldn't alarm the new mother, Carolyn confirmed my original suspicion when she said, "We have a problem. The tear goes right through into the rectum and it's going to be a pretty extensive repair. I'm not sure I'm comfortable doing it. I've never done one this big." I was impressed that Carolyn could so easily state her own limitations.

Kathryn had what we call a fourth-degree tear. Because she had started her labor with castor oil, she was still having runs of watery diarrhea, which complicated the situation. "I don't know if we can handle it here. We may have to figure out a way to get her into town," Carolyn said.

We stood silent while we all considered that possibility, listening to the rain pounding on the little cabin's roof. For a moment the rain was the only sound we heard. I was thinking furiously. My training at the hospital had taught me how to sew a fourth-degree tear. I had done a few, but always with someone else to help me. Could I do it here, without the nurses? Should I? I was only supposed to observe; my instructions had been clear. Thinking of an essential surgical instrument I would need, I tentatively asked, "Do you happen to have a Gelpi retractor in any of your kits?"

The two midwives looked at each other and then back at me. Suzette hesitated, and then said, "I do have one, but I've never used it. It was given to me and I always carry it but I don't know why."

Taking a deep breath, I made the leap. "If you have a Gelpi, I can repair a fourth-degree tear." The two of them were so excited about digging out the Gelpi that neither of them saw my trepidation. Even as I spoke, I knew I was breaking my agreement to remain an impartial observer at this birth. But my hospital training as a family practice physician had taught me how to fix a fourth-degree tear, and that is exactly what Kathryn needed.

Kathryn wanted to go to the bathroom, so we helped her walk in and sit. It wasn't long until she felt nauseated and faint, so as soon as we had her room cleaned and ready for her again we helped her back to bed. Then I got to work. I perched on the side of the bed, leaning on one elbow while the midwives held a flashlight for me to sew by. Layer by layer, I sutured the torn tissue with countless tiny stitches. Kathryn lay on her back, propped up on pillows, and patiently allowed me to sew her bottom together while she cuddled her newborn son. There were many moments that I wished for better lighting and for a good surgical table and stool to save my back, but we used what we had and made it work. We kept the area as sterile as possible, stopping frequently to change the draping. The rain continued to pound steadily on the roof overhead. Forty-five minutes later, my back was sore, my arms were all but numb, and I was sweating and exhausted, but Kathryn's bottom was neatly put back together and all the bleeding had stopped.

I moved away from the bed and let the midwives take over again while I paced, shaking my arms out and loosening up my back. Kathryn looked pretty pale to me, but Suzette said, "Your lookin' good girl! Good pulse. Let me check your blood pressure now." The two midwives were perched on either side of her bed, checking her out and helping her breastfeed, so I made my way into the kitchen to get some juice. When I came back in to offer Kathryn the juice, she shook her head, saying, "Maybe in a few minutes. I want to get him on the other breast first." She was happy and comfortable just lying in bed, resting and nursing and gazing into the face of her newborn son. I drank the juice.

The rain had finally stopped when dawn broke two hours later. The midwives were ready to make their way home. Kathryn was tucked in a clean bed eating toast and soup with her baby cuddled next to her. I looked for Maggie and realized she had fallen asleep sometime after the suturing. She was now sprawled across her little bed in the far corner of the bedroom. Next to the bed was her dollhouse. When I looked at it closely, I realized I was looking at a birthing scene Maggie had created before falling asleep. The big mommy doll was lying on a bed in the center with all the other available dolls of all sizes and shapes standing around the bed helping out.

This was not an easy delivery for anyone. I saw bravery in Kathryn and in her midwives as they all valiantly persevered through the pushing stage. We used every technique we could think of to help. More than once, I thought about the vacuum extractor, IV, instruments, and lighting available at the hospital just twenty miles away. At times it felt like we were flying by the seats of our pants and luck was with us. With a cord wrapped four times around the baby's neck and a tight fit, we needed every bit of Kathryn's determination and Carolyn's skill to pull it off. The fact that she had no help from hospital technology gave Kathryn the motivation to hang in there and keep working as hard as she did. She needed all her bravery and determination and help from her family and the midwives to stay at home. I know things would have been very different in the hospital, and not necessarily better from Kathryn's point of view.

About a year later I ran into Carolyn, the midwife who had delivered Kathryn's baby. I asked if Kathryn had recovered well, if she had any infection or any problems from the repair I had done, and how the baby was. Carolyn reported that everyone was healthy, happy, and still very satisfied with the birth experience. I breathed a huge sigh of relief. Every woman has a right to decide where and how she wants to give birth, but if she chooses a situation without access to advanced medical care, she must be willing to live with the consequences. Kathryn had done exactly what she needed to.

Retelling this birth story many years later, I am still in awe of our bravery and that this birth had such a happy ending. Years ago, I had delivered my own daughter at home with the help of midwives. After Kathryn's birthing experience, I started to consider more carefully the options we have: to birth babies at home, to birth at birthing centers, or to birth in hospitals. I thought about the risks and advantages of birthing in the comfort and safety of home and about the advantages of all the life-saving technology available in the hospital.

Home is a wonderful place to birth. If the pregnancy and labor are low risk, if the family is sincerely comfortable birthing a baby in their home, if the midwives are skilled and know when they need help, and if the home is no further than fifteen minutes from a hospital, home is an ideal place to have a baby. But if the home is too far away from life-saving technology, or if the midwives are too inexperienced or afraid to ask for help, homebirth can be a dangerous gamble.

Once I had a true appreciation of the benefits that both midwifery and hospitals bring to the birthing process, and a passion for balancing the options, I was on my way to practicing integrative childbirth.

*

I became a doctor so that I could deliver babies. But the delivery alone was never going to be enough. I also wanted to take care of the mothers before and after they were pregnant. I wanted to take care of the babies I delivered and watch them grow. I wanted to know the fathers and include them in the birth of their children. I wanted to help the grandparents through the inevitable challenges of aging. I wanted to help families when someone died. I was greedy. I wanted in on the whole life path; I didn't want to miss a single miracle. I had good reasons to be that way.

In 1949, my mother was two weeks overdue with me, her second baby. Giving birth the first time had been ridiculously simple. She remembered little of it because the whole event was clouded by the medications they used in 1947 to make birth tolerable for mothers and doctors alike. Birth seemed so easy to Mom, she thought she would have lots of children. My father, a career naval officer, had been away at sea during the first birth and so it seemed incredibly easy to him too. They had no idea what was coming.

When Mom was ready to have me, she started bleeding heavily. Despite being way past her due date, she was not prepared for things to go wrong. She and my father charged over to the Navy hospital and expected to be rescued. But on that October day in Pensacola, Florida there were no medical doctors to be found. As difficult as it is to imagine, a dentist was the closest they could find, and he was not in the least prepared for this type of emergency. My mother continued to bleed, my father wished he was back at sea in blissful ignorance of female problems, and I waited to be evicted from my mother's womb.

I have always been cautious about making up my mind, but once I decide what it is I need to do, I waste no time before acting on my decisions. Family legend has it that I saved both our lives that day. I descended into my mother's pelvis, using my hard head to stop my mother's bleeding, and barreled my way out into the world. So it was that my first action on this planet was to assist in my own birth.

I spent my childhood looking for magic. I would find it in books, in the woods, alongside creeks, and when talking to animals. Like most Navy families, we moved every two years or so, and I had no friendships that lasted longer than a year or two. I grew up alone. I was a child who loved nature, and I knew in my heart that magic was real. Everywhere we moved I would find a nearby creek where I could watch tadpoles turning into frogs, secret gardens full of caterpillars and cocoons becoming butterflies, and forests with broken eggshells—evidence of the baby birds that were hatching high above my head. Magic provided the color in my world, and the possibility that *anything* could happen. Mother Nature provided divine order; she was the unseen force that made the world turn and the seasons change. I found peace when I was close to Mother Nature. I trusted her.

During the 1970s, I was in my twenties, still hungry for experience. It was a life affected by the social upheavals of the era: the Vietnam War, the free speech movement, and the alternative-lifestyle experiments. I taught emotionally disturbed adolescents in Missouri, I taught elementary school in Tennessee, and I worked in a tomato cannery in California. I bought a school bus and taught myself enough carpentry to make my bus into a snug little home on wheels. I traveled the United States and lived in communes from Florida to Missouri to Tennessee. I married and started to create my own family.

In those adventurous years I gave birth twice. My first baby was born in a small birthing clinic in the Ozarks of southern Missouri. At that time I figured birth was a normal event that could occasionally go wrong, so I had a doctor deliver my daughter in a clinic where they could handle an emergency but where I could go home right away if all was normal. I still trusted Mother Nature but knew that she sometimes needed help. I was not going to put myself or my baby at risk by refusing help. I was lucky. I didn't need a bit of technology's help to birth that baby. My second baby was born in the woods of Tennessee by the light of the fire in our woodstove, caught by trained midwives. I was lucky. Again. And I found in birth the magic I had loved since I was a child.

I absolutely love the process of giving birth. Heck, if it hadn't been for the nine months of exhausting pregnancy and the lifetime of care each child demands, I would have given birth a dozen times. The energy at life's transitions—either birth or death—is awesome. It did not scare me. It was exhilarating. I loved the feeling of *having* to give up control to my old friend Mother Nature and allowing that force to flow through my body, which was doing its best to make the magic of a newborn baby come into the world. In most other parts of my life, I was used to taking control, but birth was bigger than me. Birth was about feeling God within me, and getting out of Her way. It was the ultimate high.

From 1973 to 1983, I lived on The Farm, an intentional spiritual community in Summertown, Tennessee. On The Farm I was taught to honor the art and skill of spiritual midwifery. Most members of this community were young and building families. At its height in the early 1980s, The Farm had a population of fifteen hundred people, almost all of them of childbearing age. As a community, we did not sanction abortion and made an offer to anyone considering this option: "Don't have an abortion. You can come to The Farm and we'll deliver your baby and take care of it, and if you ever decide you want your baby back, you can have it."

Babies were being born all the time. The word would go out on The Farm, "Monica is having her baby today!" and the whole community would buzz with excitement about this great event. The news would travel like wildfire across the multi-party line of our phone system, through the Laundromat, and down the ridges into the households. "A baby is coming today! Wonderful!" Birth always came with positive anticipation; it never occurred to us to worry about the outcome or wonder if something would go wrong. Our births almost always went well, and the midwives managed each one with a grace we honored and respected.

The midwives on The Farm delivered most babies in their homes, and the birthing statistics were phenomenal. Out of 1,917 births, the Cesarean rate was only 1.8 percent. Reviewing all the statistics from those births, it is clear that spiritual midwifery on The Farm was safe medicine. In her book *Spiritual Midwifery,* Ina May Gaskin, the founder and director of The Farm Midwifery Center, writes:

We have found that there are laws as constant as the laws of physics, electricity, or astronomy, whose influence on the progress of the birthing cannot be ignored. The midwife or doctor attending births must be flexible enough to discover the way these laws work and learn how to work within them. Pregnant and birthing mothers are elemental forces, in the same sense that gravity, thunderstorms, earthquakes, and hurricanes are elemental forces. In order to understand the laws of their energy flow, you have to love and respect them for their magnificence at the same time that you study them with the accuracy of a true scientist.

A midwife or obstetrician needs to understand about how the energy of childbirth flows—to not know is to be like a physicist who doesn't understand about gravity.

In 1983, I knew I wanted to become a physician. I wanted to be able to use what I had learned after three decades of life's lessons and spiritual searching; I could combine those lessons with the science of medicine. I did not want to limit myself to midwifery; I wanted to care for the whole family. As Ina May suggests, I wanted to respect the magnificence of each individual patient while studying him or her with the accuracy of a scientist. I had finally found what I wanted to be when I grew up: a spiritual physician. I could experience the miracle of birth and death and all that comes in between.

Things moved quickly. After two years of pre-med classes, I started medical school at the University of California at Davis in September of 1985. I was thirty-five, and I was on my way to becoming a doctor.

Four years of medical school later, I still knew I wanted to be a family physician. My vision of a spiritual physician had not wavered, but the lessons I had learned on The Farm in Tennessee were being diluted and overwhelmed by the high-tech science of a university system. I went to lectures, I took notes, I studied with my classmates, and I learned the sciences. At the end of medical school, my family and I moved from Davis to Santa Rosa so I could start my postgraduate training. This training would allow me to be a board-certified family physician. By 1989, I was finally providing care to my own patients, and although I was delivering babies, I felt dissatisfied. I knew something was missing.

I was losing my ability to see birthing as a normal event, a spiritual event, and powerful, good fun. As a resident physician, I was all too familiar with hospitals. I spent endless days and nights there, and I knew every nook and cranny and every private place I could go to catch a nap. I knew and trusted the staff and I felt at home at the Santa Rosa Community Hospital. I knew the philosophy, I knew the massive amounts of equipment and technology available to me, and I knew I was expected to use it all. I became dependent on that environment, fulfilling the expectations of my teachers and patients alike. When I worked in obstetrics, my work was full of fetal monitors, procedures, medications, life-saving resuscitation techniques, and surgeries. I soaked it all up; I knew these skills could some day save someone I loved.

But practicing medicine in a hospital was overpowering my faith in Mother Nature. I was good at stitching up torn tissue, but I agonized over my abilities to assist a delivery so there would be no need for suturing. I was learning to support the stretching perineum during labor, but I was also trying to learn to keep my hands off and avoid unnecessary or possibly harmful intervention.

My attending obstetric teachers had taught me patience—how to trust the birth process and allow the baby to stretch the mother's tissue enough to allow safe passage. They had taught me to be an excellent assistant in the operating room when C-sections were necessary. I had even quickly and safely delivered a little footling breech boy just minutes before the nurses were ready to wheel the mother away for a C-section. But I needed to balance my new knowledge with my old priorities. I missed the feeling of normal birth, the trust that the birthing process would occur without technology, and the time-tested techniques that help women birth naturally.

And so it was that I went back to midwives to find the balance.

❋

Finally, the long years of schooling and training were done and it was time for me to start a practice of my own. While the MD degree gave me the freedom to develop my own style, it also restricted me. If I was to remain a part of the established medical community, I would have to deliver babies in hospitals and not in homes. Otherwise, my malpractice insurance would not cover me.

I *wanted* to practice within the established medical community. I liked creating my own distinctive role in a community of family physicians, specialists, hospitals, and birthing centers. I enjoyed the camaraderie and respect of my peers and the stimulating medical discussions we had as we shared stories of patient encounters and challenging diagnoses. And in my own unique way, I wanted to offer compassionate and comprehensive care to patients who had restrictive insurance plans or Medicaid and could not afford to pay for boutique medicine.

So I resolved to provide hospital care that was as close to midwifery as possible. I vowed to trust Mother Nature, watch with vigilance for signs of distress, and respect each mother who honored me with her trust. I worked to integrate the midwifery model and the medical model into each birth I attended.

The first chapter in this book is written for those who will be delivering in a hospital but still want the satisfaction and empowerment of a homebirth. I define integrative childbirth and explore the five key elements necessary to prepare for this approach to birth. The birth stories that follow illustrate these five elements and show that every birth is as unique as is each child being born. Following the last birth story is a chapter written for my fellow physicians, describing a style of practice that is not only personally fulfilling, but also quite doable even in today's health care system. Everyone will enjoy the stories, but parents and professionals may want to read both the first and the last chapters, thereby gaining a point of view that can help them work together to minimize fear and put technology where it belongs.

The stories were collected over fifteen years of practicing integrative childbirth. Some births needed no intervention and were well managed by Mother Nature. These were powerful experiences, and it was a thrill to stand back and let Nature take her course. Other births required the use of medical technology, but I never ignored the mother-baby spiritual connection.

All of the births were attended by a physician, which was not always me. None occurred at home. Because these births occurred in the hospital, the reader may expect to read about the medical model: women continuously monitored with restrictive technology, episiotomies given regardless of need, and protocols turning a magnificent experience into a medical procedure. This is what our society has come to expect from hospital births managed by doctors. But instead, you will see in these births that the partnership between the provider and the laboring mother is the foundation of trust for each delivery, and that this relationship does not weaken in the heat of the moment. Rather, it becomes stronger when the births are difficult. Protocols are kept in their place, and the physician supports the woman and her family as a midwife would if they were birthing at home. And although not every story is a perfect example of an integrative childbirth, each one is an opportunity to learn. With this in mind, I have added comments to point out how sometimes things could have been managed differently to provide a better experience for the mother or the baby, as well as to emphasize learning points when things go well.

It was no surprise that I could find many women willing to tell their tales. What was surprising was that as I wrote each story's introduction, there was simply *not* an irrelevant or boring story in the whole collection. Each one is special. Each one is dramatic and suspenseful. In these stories you will find joy, triumph, sadness, frustration, surprise, humor, insight, and courage.

Birth stories can be scary, but it's the same kind of fear we have on a roller coaster ride, with its ups and downs, and we have the same exhilarating sense of relief when it's over. Most of the stories are told in the words of the women who gave birth, but some include the words of fathers, partners, and doulas (labor assistants). I've told my story first, added a bit of narration to a few, and told one from my point of view to complement the mother's version of the same tale. But the stories truly belong to the women who birthed their babies.

On behalf of all these women, their partners, the doulas who supported them, and the care providers who still understand the power of Mother Nature, I invite you to enjoy this book that honors the spirit of integrative childbirth.

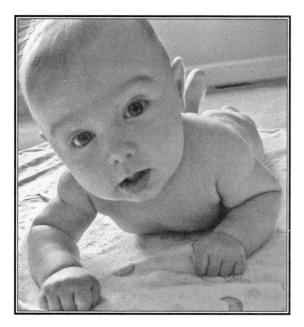

HOMEBIRTH IN THE HOSPITAL –
MAKING IT HAPPEN

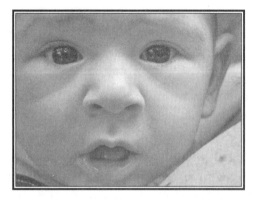

Normal birth is not a medical procedure. Normal birth is a miraculous and sometimes stressful time for families, but it usually does not require medical intervention. In reality, we find that the more we intervene in an uncomplicated birth, the more we end up taking over for Mother Nature, and all too often when we start down that slippery slope, we end up with Cesarean sections.

As a physician who has delivered many babies, I believe that normal birth is best accomplished when removed from hospital facilities full of illness, arbitrary schedules, strict protocols, and medical management. Statistics show that low-risk pregnancies are much less likely to have nonsurgical deliveries if they occur outside a hospital. Hospital births in America are currently performed by Cesarean section more than thirty percent of the time, but planned out-of-hospital births have a Cesarean section rate of only four percent.[1]

That said, the most common place for a woman to have her baby in America today is in a hospital. In part, that's due to insurance requirements and financial restrictions. Most insurance plans will not pay for a homebirth with a midwife, although many do pay for care at a birth center. Many

1   BMJ 2005;330:1416 (18 June), doi:10.1136/bmj.330.7505.1416

doctors cannot attend homebirths because their malpractice insurance restricts them to hospital practice. Some families don't want the "mess" of a birth in their home, some want to have medical help immediately available if needed, and some complications are best managed with hospital deliveries. Most American women still feel safest having their babies in hospitals.

Natural childbirth is not for everyone. Some women would give a year's salary just to have an epidural as soon as they go into labor, and others schedule elective C-sections because they fear childbirth and would like to schedule birth predictably into their busy lives. Our society supports choice, and many women take advantage of medically managed births. But something truly valuable is lost when women avoid natural childbirth.

The hormones that accompany natural childbirth are powerful, each working at the right time for the needs of the moment. During the first stages of labor, prostaglandins prepare the cervix, softening it and starting dilation. Oxytocin causes the uterus to contract. Labor also causes women to release endorphins, those same hormones that give athletes a runner's high. Endorphins are natural opiates that block pain receptors, and although they do not make labor painless, they do make it more bearable.

Immediately after a vaginal birth, oxytocin rises, stimulating the bonding that is so important to mothers and newborns. Many times I have watched a woman's face change in mere seconds—from the sweaty, sometimes frantic face associated with the concentrated effort of pushing into a relaxed and captivated Madonna reveling in her child. This is a miracle that is a byproduct of surging oxytocin.

The medical management of birth in hospitals can make a woman distrust her body's natural abilities. Fear can inhibit the release of helpful hormones, delaying or stopping labor altogether. Sadly, overriding natural hormones unnecessarily robs a mother of the help that nature provides during the hard work of having babies.

Natural childbirth also brings some surprising long-term benefits to couples, preparing them for the lifelong task of parenting. Guiding a child to maturity takes patience, perseverance, bravery, wisdom, acceptance of loss of control, humor, respect for your partner, and a lot of faith. And these exact qualities are what sustain and guide you through childbirth. So childbirth as nature intended it is a gift, teaching many of the skills parents will need through the challenges of the next twenty or thirty years.

THE DEFINITION OF INTEGRATIVE CHILDBIRTH

Integrative childbirth combines the midwifery model of care with the medical model of care.

As stated by the Midwifery Task Force in 1996, "The midwifery model of care is based on the assumption that pregnancy and birth are normal life events. This model of care includes monitoring the physical, psychological, and social well-being of the mother throughout the childbearing cycle; providing the mother with individualized education, counseling, and prenatal care, continuous hands-on assistance during labor and delivery, and postpartum support; minimizing technological interventions; and identifying and referring women who require obstetrical attention. The application of this woman-centered model has been proven to reduce the incidence of birth injury, trauma, and cesarean section."

The medical model of maternity care, in its purest form, sees pregnancy and labor as abnormal physical conditions, which must be treated with medical technology. Medical intervention is an integral part of every birth, and birth is never considered a safe process. Women's labors and deliveries are expected to fit within statistical expectations, and any deviation from these expectations is a cause for concern. Mind and body are seen as separate entities. Managing the physical aspects of birth with aggressive technology is considered appropriate medical care. Pain medication and anesthesia are offered and encouraged because the pains of childbirth are considered unnecessarily grueling.

If we combine the two styles, basing our initial care plan on the midwifery model and using medical technology only when necessary to save lives and to serve the needs of laboring mothers, we have a true integration: the best of both worlds.

The integrative childbirth model increases patient safety and decreases the physician's risk of liability by creating a strong focus on the individual and her family. Clear communication decreases the risk of litigation by improving patient satisfaction and involving patients in their own care.

It is important to remember that *technology should never replace experienced human attention* during the birthing process.

When the midwifery model is applied, between eighty-five and ninety-five percent of healthy women will safely give birth without surgery or the use of instruments. Medical interventions come into play as part of sensible monitoring during pregnancy, labor, and delivery, but only if they're clearly necessary. In reality, intervention is often inappropriate and may actually be harmful when used purely for convenience or profit.

To facilitate an integrative childbirth, it is essential to make plans ahead of time. Once you go into labor, your ability to control the situation is severely limited. Throughout your labor and delivery, you want to feel safe, without having to negotiate the details. You cannot control the natural labor process, but you can control the planning and choices you make. You have that right, and the right to deliver your child without disappointment or regrets.

＊

Let's consider five key elements to a successful integrative birth—I call them the Five Cs: Choice, Communication, Continuity, Confidence, and Control of Protocols.

CHOICE

Assume your pregnancy, your health, and your baby's health are all normal. Your pregnancy is considered low risk, without any anticipated needs for medical intervention. You get to choose your provider and the facility you want to go to for your delivery. These choices may be limited by financial constraints or insurance requirements, but the final decision is yours.

Which provider will you choose to be the guardian of your safety? You can go to obstetrics and gynecology (ob/gyn) specialist, a family physician, or a midwife for your prenatal care and delivery. Obstetric gynecologists are surgeons and usually more technologically oriented than family physicians. You are likely to have some kind of medical intervention if you choose to work with an ob/gyn doctor, even if it's just continuous monitoring or a precautionary IV. Family physicians can practice like specialists, like midwives, or anywhere in between. Some family doctors have hospital privileges for Cesarean sections, are most comfortable using the medical model, and adhere to strict protocols. Some practice very much like midwives, with personalized care and minimal intervention.

Family physicians can come with you to the operating room and assist the specialist if a Cesarean section is necessary. Lastly, midwives with hospital privileges can manage your labor and deliver your baby in the hospital, and they are most likely (but not always) willing to forego medical interventions. However, they cannot go to surgery, and your care will transfer to the backup surgeon if surgery becomes necessary.

Only careful interviews with individual providers can help you identify their style of practice. When you interview physicians, ask them for their Cesarean-section rate for the previous year of practice. You may refer to the checklist at the end of this chapter for other questions to consider during your interviews, but the C-section rate may be the single most important piece of information you will need.

Women in labor need a lot of emotional encouragement and it is unrealistic to expect your physician or the hospital staff to be your main source of support. This support needs to be consistently positive; anxious, nervous, and fearful friends can actually obstruct the birth process. Your partner is usually the one expected to fill this need, but often it takes more than one person. Consider inviting a professional doula to be your labor attendant or asking a trusted family member to provide support so that you are never alone while you are in labor. By carefully choosing your attendants based on referrals and personal interviews, you can create a birth team that works well together.

Listen to others who have *good* birth stories to tell and ask them where their babies were born. Women will be quick to tell you about their wonderful providers, but be careful about choosing a situation just because someone says it was fantastic for her or someone she knows. Ask direct questions (see the checklist at the end of this chapter), and make sure you are comfortable with the answers you get. What worked for your sister or your friend may not be the best choice for you.

Your choice of hospital is as important as your choice of provider. Different hospitals support very different styles of birth. Some will be more supportive of integrative childbirth; others will adhere more closely to a medical model. The birth culture created by the medical staff will vary as well.

A labor and delivery unit staffed primarily by ob/gyn doctors is more likely to manage births medically. Ob/gyn doctors are skilled surgeons— exactly who you want around when you need a surgical solution to a life-threatening complication. But many, perhaps even most ob/gyn doctors, have never seen a natural childbirth. The nurses working in these hospitals are comfortable with IVs, Pitocin, pain medications, and other medical interventions. They're trained to use those interventions and may be anxious if they can't use the technology available to them.

Hospitals staffed primarily by midwives and family physicians are usually more comfortable with integrative birth. Midwives have seen many natural births and have learned to trust the process. The majority of family physicians want to encourage vaginal deliveries, so they may be more willing to work with a woman in a protracted labor, whereas a specialist would call for surgery more quickly. The nursing staff at hospitals that support natural births may be less quick to use technology and more open to alternative labor-management techniques.

Do your research. Call your local hospitals and ask for their annual Cesarean-section rates. Pay attention to the hospital's response to your request for information; when I called my own local hospitals I found that the hospital with the highest rate was the most reluctant to share their statistics. Ask if their staff includes midwives, and see if the midwives have delivery privileges; some hospitals only allow physicians to deliver babies. Even if you are not going to work with a midwife, this information will help you understand the underlying culture and attitude of a hospital. Providers in your community know the local birth culture too, so ask for their opinions and make sure the provider you choose has privileges at the facility you trust.

Remember: the choice is yours, and the time to make it is before you go into labor.

COMMUNICATION

Pregnant women usually have countless questions, especially during a first pregnancy. You have questions about everything—about the tests and procedures that are ordered, labor and delivery expectations, and every little twinge you feel in your body. Even if you've birthed before, you'll find yourself quizzing providers, friends, mothers, sisters, casual acquaintances, and unknown sources on the Internet. And even if the provider answers all your questions, everyone else will eagerly offer opinions.

In integrative childbirth, you should discuss questions and concerns with the provider as part of your prenatal care. Clear communication at each visit builds realistic expectations and provides an essential foundation for making difficult decisions, if needed, during the intensity of a birth.

Many doctors have their nurses gather and record information about each newly pregnant woman, or have the patient fill out information forms. The doctor then reviews this information later, when he has the opportunity to do paperwork and go over charts. Going over the data in this way may appear to be an efficient use of time, but it's not. I cannot overstate the importance of a woman sharing her information directly with her provider. *This is the first step to integrative childbirth.* The half-hour intake session is the beginning of a relationship you will be depending upon seven months later.

If your provider doesn't get to know you well, she will be inclined to depersonalize your care in the hospital, relying primarily on monitors to assess your situation. Trust and open communication cannot be created without taking the time to talk. During one of your initial visits, you should be able to discuss your past medical history, your family support, possible religious limitations, and any other issues that might affect your pregnancy. The provider should get a sense of how you and your partner work together, how you solve problems, and how your individual personalities interact.

Early in your relationship, the provider should clearly explain her style of care. If she offers something different than what you expect, you should find a more suitable situation sooner rather than later. Look for hands-on watchfulness, which means that the provider supports you while Mother Nature does her work. The care provider should watch with vigilance but without unnecessary interference and should address issues immediately as the need arises. Don't confuse "natural" with lack of care. A medical doctor has a responsibility to provide a certain standard of care to decrease your risks and help ensure a healthy baby. You want the provider to order all the necessary lab tests, order sonograms if indicated, and explain everything she recommends.

After the first visit, you should see this same provider for a brief but focused visit once a month until your last month of pregnancy. Even fifteen minutes of a physician's *undivided* attention can feel like a half-hour of communication, and fifteen minutes is plenty of time for him to check your belly, measure it, listen to the heartbeat, and discuss your concerns. Be sure to bring a written list of questions to each appointment. For instance, you'll want to ask about necessary screening tests, whether sonograms are needed, and plans for the delivery (see checklist). A good provider will address most of these concerns before you even ask, and this is a sign that you are making a good connection.

By the ninth month, all your questions should be answered. You will have created a relationship that will enable you to trust and work well with this provider during labor and delivery. And if you are unable to communicate or have a serious incompatibility, you will have figured this out long before you go into labor.

CONTINUITY

Continuity of care is one of the primary reasons women choose midwives rather than physicians to deliver their babies. Increasingly, the physician who provides prenatal care cannot promise to be available when a woman goes into labor. Keeping up with deliveries that happen in the middle of a busy clinic day or in the middle of the night is stressful and demanding, and being on call for all deliveries is often impossible. Most often, groups of physicians share call, and no one knows who will deliver a baby until the time comes and the on-call doctor shows up. It is not only doctors who arrange call schedules—this arrangement is becoming more common among groups of midwives, too.

To have an integrative childbirth, it is important for you to know and trust the person who is delivering your baby. You will be in no position to renegotiate birth agreements while having contractions. Besides, by now you've spent several months building a relationship for the event! Ask about the other providers who may be on call when you go into labor, and make sure their philosophy and style of practice is supportive of your personal needs. The call partners need to offer the same type of delivery experience that you expect from your primary provider—one based on full communication, trust, and minimal interventions.

You have a right to meet with the call partners sometime during your pregnancy, preferably early enough to help you decide if you have made the right choice of providers. If you have not met the other physicians prior to your last month of pregnancy, take advantage of the weekly visits scheduled near your due date to speak with them. These physicians should not be strange faces appearing for the first time when you deliver.

You may find that a family physician is more flexible than an ob/gyn specialist and therefore able to personally attend your birth. Also, if a family physician delivers your baby, he can be your baby's doctor, and this seamless continuity of care is comforting. During my years of practice, I have attended most of my patients' deliveries, but there have been a few times when I needed someone to cover for me. I know I have excellent call partners when I consistently get good reports from patients about the handful of births I missed.

CONFIDENCE AND TRUST

The pregnant woman must trust her provider with her life, and with the life of her baby. You must have confidence that your provider will follow through on the agreements made during prenatal care. You should expect full communication, to be told the truth, and not to have to defend your preferences while you are in labor.

Similarly, you need to be honest and communicative with your provider throughout your pregnancy. You need to know you can voice your concerns and be heard. During the birth, with all the added stressors of nervous family members, the busy hospital staff, and the realities of labor, this trust will be the cornerstone of an integrative childbirth. Trust is built over time and will happen naturally if you have honest and open communication with your provider.

You will have made agreements about care with your provider before you go into labor. Ideally, procedures initiated during labor should be discussed and agreed upon at the time, though in the case of a sudden emergency, you must rely on your physician to act quickly and without negotiation.

Whenever I think of the trust issue, I remember a particular birth early in my career. Riki and Christine lived in the mountains and drove for more than two hours to come in for their prenatal appointments. They felt the effort was worth it because they wanted to be able to birth their baby with minimal intervention and in the hospital where they felt safe and where their insurance would cover the costs.

They were a fiercely independent couple; Christine stayed in shape throughout her pregnancy by hiking the mountains they called home. When her due date was near, they came down to stay in a hotel near the hospital to await labor. They spent her early labor in the hotel and came in to the hospital when she was almost six centimeters dilated. All went well until the second stage, when Chris started pushing. In spite of a powerful effort, this baby was not coming out. Two hours passed, then three. There was plenty of room in Christine's pelvis. We did everything we could think of, short of medical intervention: changed pushing positions, made sure the people in attendance were not getting in the way, and kept Chris hydrated. She and Riki refused anything else, and because Chris and the baby were both doing well, I allowed her to continue pushing.

Four hours passed, then five, then six. The room was feeling stale. The nurses had changed shifts, and the new energy did nothing to help Chris bring that baby further down the birth canal. Still, she and Riki refused intervention. More hours passed. The baby was doing fine, but Chris was exhausted. The nurses were starting to question my tactics. Finally I had to explain that whether she wanted it or not, Chris was going to need help getting her baby out. Even with my minimalist style of labor management, I knew that Mother Nature needed help with this one.

I suggested starting some Pitocin to stimulate the uterus and produce stronger contractions. Chris was so tired she would have done anything I said, but Riki was protecting her by questioning my suggestions. After all, Chris had said very clearly, "Don't let them give me any medicine if I can do it naturally!" As the doctor responsible for a safe birth, I saw Pitocin as a small intervention compared to the C-section most of my colleagues would have performed several hours ago. But Riki saw it as questionable.

I explained the risks of continuing along the path we were on: more pushing, more disappointing fatigue, and possibly a C-section if the baby started showing signs of distress. Riki was obviously confused and torn about what to do. Finally, I stood up tall and looked this six-foot, four-inch man in the eyes and asked him point blank, "Are you going to trust me to do what it takes to give you a healthy baby?" He searched my eyes for deception, blinked, and said, "Of course I will. Go ahead and do what it is you do best." I started a Pitocin IV drip and thirty minutes later Jacob was born—healthy and lusty—and handed to a very tired Christine. For nine months I had been building this relationship bit by bit. In the end, they had no regrets and neither did I.

CONTROL OF PROTOCOLS

A final ingredient essential to integrative childbirth is the recognition that *protocols are not people.* Had I delivered Riki and Christine's baby by hospital protocols, they would have had an invasive and, most likely, surgical delivery—long before their healthy boy was born vaginally. Being in the room with the family and watching the baby's heart rate myself allowed me to override hospital protocol and provide a safe vaginal birth experience in accordance with the mother's wishes. I was watching people, not protocols.

Prenatal management is full of protocols. Physicians spend hours in committees creating extensive lists of recommended rules for managing pregnancy, labor, and delivery. The recommendations are based on experience, statistical risk factors, and current studies on pregnant women. Some are based completely on malpractice and litigation fears. Certain tests are done at certain times, fetal ultrasounds may be ordered routinely, and IVs and fetal monitors may be automatically inserted when women arrive at the hospital. Some of these protocols make sense and are not only valid, but essential, for quality care; others are specific to situations that affect a minority of women. But individual women may not want to be managed by protocols that are not dictated by their individual needs or preferences.

The most common way a laboring woman loses power is by being given homogenous care based on hospital protocols. The continuous use of monitors, rigid expectations of a time line for labor, use of medications—all these may not be necessary for the individual laboring woman. To have an integrative birth, you'll want to choose a physician who promises to consider you as an individual with unique labor needs.

Your provider should be your advocate in the hospital, ordering only those procedures that are necessary to your unique situation. You and she should discuss ahead of time the hospital's protocols and procedures so that you know what to expect. Of course, it is important for the staff to have enough freedom to provide a safe birth. If trust is established, a birthing woman should be comfortable accepting the need for some protocols.

The fear of protocols and the resulting loss of control leads people to create their own birth plan—their own set of personal rules and expectations. Birth plans are wonderful as a way to consider your options and express your needs, but they need to be taken with a grain of salt. Many physicians laugh or roll their eyes when presented with a birth plan, because they know how rapidly things change during a labor and delivery. But birth plans are an important form of communication and should be taken seriously for that reason alone. If you decide to write a birth plan, sometime in the last month of prenatal care you and your physician should review it, discuss any differences of opinion, and agree on realistic goals.

For example, many women say they do not want to be strapped to a fetal monitor while they are in labor and want to know if they can refuse to be monitored. Fetal monitors do restrict mobility, and I happen to agree that it is not good for a normal laboring woman to be immobilized by technology. In fact, research has shown that continuous monitoring does not improve outcomes and often leads to unnecessary interventions. On the other hand, I do want to be able to periodically check the fetal heart rate.

Most often, a pregnant woman and I will agree to an initial fifteen-minute monitor check (for everyone's reassurance on admission) and then brief periodic checks thereafter as long as things are going well. If I honor a mother's need to labor freely and she honors her caregivers' need to know that her baby appears well, we arrive at a plan that assures everyone's well-being. Hospital protocol is satisfied, the staff is reassured, and the laboring mother keeps her mobility.

We have a saying in my practice: "Burn the birth plan!" My patients were the ones who coined this phrase when they realized during their labors that Mother Nature had her own ideas. They knew a change of plans was always a possibility, and I'm sure to emphasize this fact in our discussions. Rigid attachment to any birth scenario is not helpful to either the laboring mother or to her caregivers, and the initial discussion of birth plans is the perfect time to talk about accepting the course of a natural birth.

Every woman has a unique birth story. With the right planning, your experience can include the compassionate providers and personal empowerment usually associated with a homebirth, even if you are birthing in a hospital. Do your research and find an experienced provider who will develop a personal relationship with you and who will safely support you during a delivery, no matter what surprises Mother Nature has in store. Make sure that everyone on your team—your provider, the nurses, and your support crew—all have faith in the birthing process and your ability to birth your baby without unnecessary interventions. Most of all, have faith in yourself. Allow your body to do what it does well, and you will have an empowering birth story to share for generations to come.

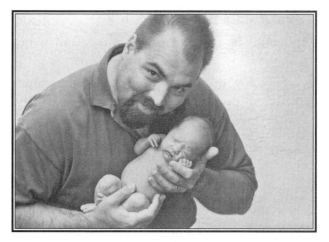

CHECKLIST FOR EVALUATING INTEGRATIVE CHILDBIRTH PROVIDERS

❏ Who performs the intake interviews, gathers the initial patient/client information, and does the first thorough physical exam?

❏ How much time does the initial visit take?

❏ Who will you see for your subsequent prenatal visits?

❏ Does each visit include a blood pressure check, weight check, urine check, belly measurement, and a fetal heartbeat check? Do you get to hear the heartbeat, too?

❏ Can you eat and drink while you're in labor?

❏ How often does the provider cut an episiotomy?

❏ Do you have to be moved from a labor room to a delivery room to have your baby?

❏ Assuming a normal birth, is your baby given to you immediately?

❏ What is the Cesarean-section rate in the provider's practice?

❏ Do they have automatic protocols, such as:

   ❏ Checking your cervix weekly after a certain date?

   ❏ Sonograms at regular intervals?

   ❏ Induction by a certain date or immediately when your water breaks?

❏ Who will deliver your baby when you go into labor?

   ❏ If there is a call group, are the other members supportive of integrative childbirth?

   ❏ Can you meet the other providers before you go into labor?

❏ Where does the provider deliver babies?

   If it's in a hospital:

   ❏ Is the hospital staff supportive of integrative childbirth?

   ❏ What is the hospital's C-section rate?

   ❏ Are protocols negotiable?

   ❏ Do they take your insurance for payment?

If it's in a birth center:

❏ How far are they from the hospital?

❏ What are the criteria for transfer to a hospital?

❏ Do they have a good working relationship with the hospital staff?

❏ Do they take your insurance for payment? Does their backup hospital take your insurance?

❏ Does the provider's style of care reasonably match your needs?

❏ Are you able to clearly communicate with the provider?

❏ Do you trust the provider?

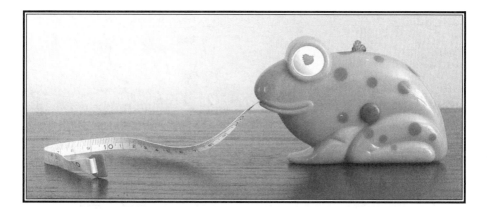

A Woman's Will

Stacey and Sarah Kate

Although it has been over thirty years since my first child was born, I remember it like it was yesterday. Unlike my mother, I was given no medication, but that didn't keep the event from being surreal. This was not a homebirth, but it was medically supported. I found that going to a birth center in 1973 was as close as I could get to a homebirth in a hospital.

Don and I were living in the woods of central Missouri, just north of the Ozarks, in a county of green rolling hills and slow muddy waters. We were part of a spiritual community of approximately twenty people, but only about eight of us actually lived on the property. The rest lived and worked in town. Out on the farm we had no electricity and no indoor plumbing, and we hauled our water in a bucket from an old cistern of fresh rainwater collected in the front yard. Bath water was heated on a propane stove. Kerosene lamps provided light, but we usually went to sleep shortly after dark and woke with the dawn.

I quit my teaching job when I got pregnant, so I had plenty of time to keep the wood fires stoked and prepare for the baby that would be born in the spring. Several friends of mine had already had babies, so I figured I could do it, too. I learned about pregnancy and labor by reading an old, orange paperback I found that may have been the first Bradley book; I can't remember.

I was interested only in the birthing process. Specific techniques for managing labor didn't seem important to me. I figured I would rise to the occasion when I needed to. Long before I ever considered becoming a doctor and delivering babies for others, I trusted Mother Nature to take care of me. I was still young enough to know how to get out of her way and wise enough to accept all the loving support I was offered.

Most of us hold the memory of our children's births clearly in our minds. It is one of those life-changing events that are burned in our minds and hearts forever. Here is the story I remember.

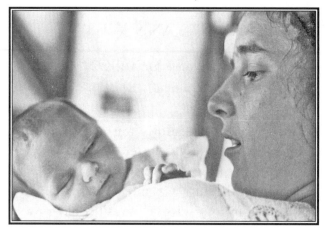

Stacey and her newborn

It was 1973 and I was very young. Maybe not young by some standards, but I knew very little and trusted so much. I was twenty-three. When I was pregnant, I saw no reason to go to a hospital for delivery. As a matter of fact, I saw many reasons to stay away from hospitals. When I went to the local hospital to check it out, I was told that after delivery, my baby would be put in a nursery. The only way I could keep my baby near me was by giving birth outside the hospital so that it was "contaminated" when we came in; they couldn't allow a baby contaminated by the world outside to be around the babies in the hospital nursery. If that policy was any indication of their health care philosophy, I wanted no part of it. Those were the days of natural childbirth. People were having their babies at home, with friends assisting in the deliveries, and many of us were rejecting the status quo.

I had considered traveling to Tennessee to have my baby on The Farm where midwives would care for me in a supportive community, but travel didn't sound like a good idea. I was not brave or foolish enough to birth alone in the woods. This was my first baby, and I had no idea how much help I might need. I wanted support, but not unnecessary interference. So I searched.

About sixty miles south of our little farm was a doctor who would deliver my baby in a birthing clinic, and if all was well, we could go home a couple of hours after the birth. I knew a couple of other women who had gone to this doctor and they assured me that he would be the perfect choice. If we needed something drastic like a C-section, he had privileges at a good hospital nearby. After meeting him, I decided to be safe and deliver at Dr. Howard's clinic.

Throughout my pregnancy, I traveled sixty miles each way for my prenatal checkups. I was not a happy pregnant person. In fact, I was miserable. I never recovered from the nausea of early pregnancy because I never figured out that eating was what made the nausea go away. I rarely ate. Fried potatoes were the only food that appealed to me. One afternoon, Don brought me a full gallon of ice cold whole milk, bought fresh that morning from the farmer down the road. It looked wonderful, and I downed at least a quart in one sitting. It went down like the elixir of life and I knew then that I must have been severely malnourished. But I was young and seemed healthy in spite of my diet. My doctor apparently didn't notice that I was not eating. At each visit he would say that all was well.

My due date was May 7th, and the evening of the 9th I was lying in bed ready to go to sleep. Don was downstairs talking to his parents on the phone, trying to explain why the baby hadn't come yet. They lived in California, and I'm sure they had strong doubts about our back-to-the-land lifestyle. They were worried. It was then that I felt my first contraction.

Don came upstairs and stretched out on the bed beside me. I lay next to him, waiting to see if the contractions were going to continue. When I felt certain they were real enough to take seriously, I told him I thought maybe something was starting to happen. Neither of us knew what that something might be, so we called our friend Patricia over to our room. Patricia, her husband, and their two kids had already settled in for the night in their room across the hall from ours. She was experienced, had already had two babies, knew how it was supposed to feel, and was planning to come along to help us with our birthing.

Smiling in anticipation, she came over to my bed, gently putting her hand on my belly. I asked her if this was how it was supposed to be. After feeling a contraction tighten the mound that was my belly, she assured me that this was definitely the real thing. So I waddled down the stairs to the kitchen and called Dr. Howard to tell him what was up. I expected him to tell me to wait awhile and see if things progressed, but he took my every-seven-to-ten-minute contractions seriously. He ordered me to get in the car and down to the clinic just as fast as I could, and if I couldn't make it that far, stop halfway down at the hospital in Jefferson City. Without much ado, the three of us got in the old white Chevy and started driving south.

The roads down into the Ozarks were narrow, dark, and winding. I was glad for the distractions of the drive, helping me take my mind off the unfamiliar sensations of labor. Sitting there in the front seat next to Don and focusing on the white line marking the edge of the two-lane highway, I was having regular, strong contractions. Patricia would reach over from the back seat occasionally and rest her hand on my belly, helping me to focus and reminding me that she was there to help. I turned to watch Don's face in the lights from the dash.

I knew Don was a skeptic. He was the sort of person who didn't believe anything he himself couldn't see or feel, so I wasn't all that surprised when he told us he didn't believe I was really in labor. It didn't matter that I couldn't reply, being busy that moment with a particularly strong contraction. However, if the doctor thought we should head south, and if Patricia assured him it was real, he was willing to humor us. It was about a half-hour after we left the farm when he looked over at me with astonishment and said, "I think I just felt a contraction!" After that he believed that it was really going to happen. I don't know what he felt, or how it felt to him, but I was past caring whether he believed me or not. I was busy.

I remember opening my eyes after being swept by a powerful contraction and seeing the headlights on the trees looming over the road. There was a deer standing on the side of the road ahead of us. She gazed at us without moving, seeming to wonder at our intrusion into her night. Nothing surprised me. I was in the middle of something far beyond my own control.

I was not in pain, but I was working hard to breathe, trying not to swirl down helplessly into the sensations overtaking my body. My belly was squeezing with a force stronger than anything I had ever felt before, and it was a force that wiped out every other sensation. During a contraction

I could hear nothing, see nothing, say nothing, and feel nothing but the strength of my womb. Then it would be over and I could open my eyes and come back to the reality of the car, the night, and the road ahead of us. There was no question about it—I had to stay right in the present moment or I would be lost. It felt like some of the good acid trips I had taken when I was in college: loss of control and altered reality, but in a very good way. I was holding on for dear life, but I wasn't scared.

We arrived at the clinic at about one o'clock in the morning. Between the car and the back door of the clinic, we had to stop three times as contractions gripped me. Standing up and walking seemed to bring on labor stronger than ever. When we reached the door, I looked up and saw Kate waiting for us—a sweet, portly nurse who quickly took us into a small room and settled me into a bed. It felt great to lie down after sitting for the last two hours and walking the distance from the car to the bed. I hadn't been there for more than a couple of minutes when Dr. Howard stepped into the room and said cheerfully, "Well! Looks like we might have a baby sometime soon!"

"Yeah," I thought. "That's an understatement." Dr. Howard did a quick check of my cervix, which didn't bother me a bit. I didn't care who did what as long as he didn't get in the way of the work I was doing.

Stepping back from the bed, Dr. Howard looked at me with raised eyebrows and said, "I don't know why you're working so hard! It's going to be another six to eight hours before this baby is born."

I thought to myself, "No *way* am I doing this for another six to eight hours! Not on your life!" My will was more focused than it had ever been. It was not conscious will, it wasn't even a logical thought, but I was absolutely certain that my labor was not going to take as long as he predicted.

I now know that I was probably four centimeters dilated when he checked me, because the estimated time from four centimeters of dilation to birth is generally six to eight hours.

I said that I wanted to go to the bathroom. The doctor and Kate looked at each other, and then said I could do that but I couldn't stay in there too long. They certainly didn't want me to deliver on the toilet.

What happened during the next little while is a blur. I remember I needed to go to the bathroom, and Patricia helped me walk to a tiny closet attached to the bedroom. The privacy of that little room was welcome for a few minutes, until the contractions strengthened and I realized I didn't want to be alone. Don was somewhere in the bedroom, but I wanted another woman by my side. I called for Patricia, made my way back to the bed, and a few minutes later felt a strong sense of pressure. This was a new and urgent sensation that was quickly overwhelming all others, so Patricia went for help, even though it had only been about fifteen minutes since they had left us alone to labor.

Kate came bustling back into the room and checked my cervix, and before I knew it I was on a gurney being wheeled down a wide hallway. Patricia and Don were jogging alongside me, keeping up with Kate. Dark windows opened to the night on one side of me, and empty quiet rooms passed by on the other. We were alone in the clinic that night.

Within minutes, I was in a brightly lit delivery room where I moved yet again onto a delivery table with big metal stirrups. I was being draped with blue sheets, and everyone seemed to be yelling at me not to push, not to push, not yet. I saw a table full of fancy metal instruments and a clear plastic box that looked like pictures I'd seen of baby incubators. Dr. Howard appeared between my knees, and after that I quit looking at anything, focused on doing the pushing that my body was demanding.

I pushed with all my strength and determination for no more than ten minutes, paying no attention to anyone or anything other than the urges of my body. I can't say I remember what it felt like when Sarah slithered out; I remember only the relief I felt when Mother Nature finally released her hold on me. Dr. Howard held up my baby so that I could see she was a girl and then tucked her into the warm little incubator. I wasn't given a chance to touch her yet, but I was able to see her curled on her belly in the incubator when they wheeled me back to my room. It did not occur to me to keep her with me.

It was an hour later when Dr. Howard walked in with my baby. I was neatly tucked

Today's homebirth in a hospital would not separate a mother from her newborn unless there was some serious medical reason to do so. In 1973, this brief separation was the norm.

back into my labor bed, chatting and laughing with Patricia and Don, reliving the high moments of the last few hours. He was holding Sarah in his arms, and she was swaddled like a little burrito. He stood at the foot of my bed, cradling her with a sweetness and reverence that showed how much he really appreciated the moment. He told me that my baby was perfect and gently lowered her into my waiting arms. He told me that I had done well, pronounced us both healthy, and said that when I felt good enough to sweep the floor, we could all go home.

Going home so quickly after an uncomplicated delivery was only possible because this occurred in a birth center. If you have your baby in a hospital, you will probably stay at least twenty-four hours to get some rest and make sure you and baby are doing well.

Two hours later, we started back north to our little farmhouse. We drove slowly, and I held my newborn in my lap the whole way—those were the days before car seats. The roads were quiet on that spring Sunday in May, and the early morning sunlight revealed beauty in a forest that had loomed dark the night before.

The next time I had a baby, I didn't bother to go anywhere. I stayed home, and the midwives came to me. Three years after our first daughter was born, we birthed Cara on The Farm in the woods of Tennessee. We labored in a one-room cabin Don had built for us, with labor attendants stoking the wood stove all night to keep the cabin warm for the coming baby. The same thing happened. I was standing during a contraction when Don looked at me and said, "It looks like this one will be born at about the same time as before."

"How much longer is that?" I gasped as soon as the contraction was over, and he said, "Oh, maybe another three hours or so." I felt a familiar confidence come over me and decided at that moment to go ahead and have this baby soon. Cara was born fifteen minutes later. *I sincerely believe that a woman's will is a force to be respected, and if there is nothing in the way of that will, miracles will happen.* I had no conscious control of my labor, but

I did encourage it and trust it. My "decisions" were not intellectual or logical; they were instinctual. I carry this lesson with me to all the births I attend: Never try to predict how quickly labor will progress. It has a life of its own, and I am humble enough to respect the power and the miracles I see each time a baby is born.

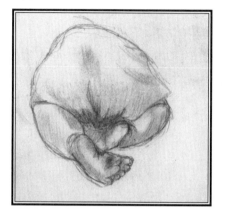 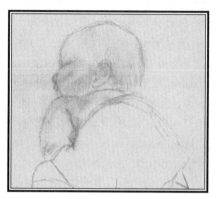

Because we had no camera, I made sketches of my perfect baby

DO WHAT YOU NEED TO DO

PAMELA AND CHLOÉ

Pamela and Peter are both used to being able to control all the big projects in their lives. Peter owns retail and wholesale stores in Marin County, California, and Pamela is an experienced project manager. Both are very good at organizing, managing, and completing projects, and they thought they could draw on these skills when they started a family. They found out, though, that their ideas about control and management had to change when dealing with Mother Nature.

Pamela was disappointed with the medically managed birth of her first child. She was determined to make her second birth one that met her expectations, one that integrated the noninvasive midwifery model with the safety and convenience of a hospital. Just because Pamela had a less-than-optimal experience the first time around didn't mean she couldn't make dreams come true the second time.

Studies have shown that women who have a labor assistant have easier labors and fewer complications. It is a sign of our times that studies must be done to prove what many women know intuitively: Birth is a community event and demands the loving and positive support of a community. Chloé's birth is a wonderful example of the healing power found in such a community.

Each pregnancy and birth is different, just as each child is different. Pamela decided to make sure this birth was different from her first by having adequate support. With the assistance of Jessica, a doula, Pamela was able to feel confident she could have the birth she wanted. When Pamela expressed her fear or doubt, Jessica helped her focus on a couple of positive thoughts, or affirmations. Pamela repeated these affirmations to herself over and over and they gave her the strength she needed to birth naturally just the way she wanted. Chloé was born in a hospital, delivered by a doctor, but with minimal medical intervention. Pamela had the integrative birth she planned, and the disappointments of the past were replaced by the joys of the present.

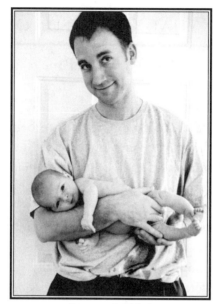

Peter and Chloé

PAMELA: Chloé is my second child. Chloé's birth story is unique because her three-year-old sister Caroline's was so stereotypical. Everything that could have gone wrong in Caroline's birth went wrong. I had a lot of ideas about how I wanted my first birth to go. I was educated, read a lot, talked to a lot of friends, and did what I thought was necessary to prepare myself. I took Lamaze and all those classes. But nobody can prepare you for giving birth.

You can't have Chloé's birth story without Caroline's because they are so interconnected. Caroline's was long. It started very early in the morning on Monday, and she wasn't born until Wednesday. I had an obstetrician at Kaiser. I also had a good friend who had had a baby at Kaiser a year prior, but she had the great knowledge to have a doula with her. She had spoken of a doula, but it sounded so foreign. And I was so silly because I thought, "Why would I want somebody I've never met before and don't know that well in the room with me while I'm having a baby?"

I had ideals. I had the birth plan that I had typed up and it was beautiful—it even had some graphics on it. I know now that doctors find this kind of detailed planning so obnoxious. I wanted no medical intervention, no epidural, and no drugs. I did not want a vacuum extraction. I wanted to breast feed immediately. These were all the normal basic wants and needs. I was under the misconception that once I got to the hospital I would be safe, that I would be cared for. I thought that my plan was all-inclusive.

But I had the opposite experience. I was not taken care of. I was ignored. I was belittled. I was criticized. I was called everything negative you can imagine by the nurse that was on duty that night. She had no patience with me. And so that just fed my fear. Everything got tense and constricted, and I wasn't dilating at all. The contractions were coming but nothing was working. My body just shut down. It was a rough start.

If you are well prepared and constantly attended by your own birth team, you will not be dependent on the hospital staff for your emotional support. The nurses on duty may not be the right ones to support you.

Of course, I had Nubain (IV pain medication), I had an epidural, and I had a vacuum extraction. She was eight pounds, four ounces, but it was only one suck and she was out. We were thankful for that. But I was on planet Wherever, and Peter and I were not connecting, which was awful. He couldn't do anything to calm me down. I vomited. I was hysterical. I was just out of it.

After I recovered, I realized that I had a beautiful, healthy baby. I was on cloud nine and proud of myself and happy and delirious and in love, but the process was not great for me.

When we got pregnant the second time, I knew I didn't want to go through that process again. And I knew that I needed to do whatever it took to make that happen. I knew Kaiser wasn't going to do it for me. And I knew I couldn't sit there and say, "Well, maybe I'll get a different nurse. Maybe I'll get a nurse that's in a good mood. Maybe I'll get a nurse who's had kids. Maybe, maybe, maybe. . ." So I said, "No I've got to prepare myself for this because I want this to be the way I know it can be. It can be a transforming, magical, empowering, enriching experience."

I still had the ideal. I didn't want medical intervention. I wanted it to be primal and tribal. I wanted to get back to the way it was supposed to be. Because I had this other voice in my head that said women have, for centuries and centuries, done this out in the woods and in the fields, and why can't I? How am I different? I did some more reading. I read a good book that had a lot of stories in it. A lot of them sounded just like my first birth story. I said, "Wow, there are a lot of people out there that had the same experience. I'm not alone. It's not because I'm weak or stupid."

The wonderful friend who had had a doula at her first birth was pregnant again. We were about eight weeks apart, and she mentioned her doula again. And this time I listened closely. I took her seriously and thought, "Hmmm. That does sound good. It doesn't seem so much like a stranger now that I know the nurses can be even more like strangers than that. If I had somebody I could meet a couple of times prior to having the baby..."

I got a few names from my friend's midwife, made some calls, and decided to feel this whole doula thing out. I was pretty sure it was going to be a good thing to have someone there just for me. It couldn't be anything but a good thing. And if I had a birth just like my birth with Caroline, so be it. At least I had someone there saying the right things and letting me know what was happening. "Okay, now you're in transition." Or, "Okay, this is the tough part." Or being the cheerleader that I so needed, the cheerleader that poor Peter had no idea how to be. I mean he was there holding my hand and loving me, but he had no idea what to do.

PETER: That's right. Those classes you take are pretty much useless once you get going. Not only that, but the dynamics of couples in situations like she was describing... Not only did I lose her, but then we had no connection. In birth courses they would tell me to encourage Pamela: "Just tell her to get up and walk around." And I'd say to her, "Get up and walk around, Pamela." There's no way. She was so far gone and so mad at the pain and everything. There's no way I was going to get her off that bed. I'm her husband and there are all those relationship dynamics coming out. "I'm not getting up. No way. Go away."

Fathers experiencing their own growing pains are not necessarily good birth attendants. Fear, anxiety, and anger can make birth more difficult by releasing adrenaline, an obstructive hormone. But if fathers take time to learn about childbirth and are fully committed to their wives and to the birth process, they can be wonderful helpmates.

PAMELA: I couldn't hear him. He couldn't reach me. It was frustrating for him. So I found Jessica and knew the minute that I spoke to her on the phone that we connected. That was important for me. I wanted to connect. I mean we didn't have to become friends—although we did become very good friends, which was a blessing—but I knew it didn't *have* to be that way. It did have to be somebody that I felt fairly comfortable with because I wanted to feel safe. She came over and met me and we hit it off. I asked her if she wanted to be my doula. She's unique in that she gave me so much of herself and so much of her time.

We met in July, and I was due in December. She came to see me at least once a month in the beginning of my pregnancy, and then she started coming every two weeks. She would come over and have tea and we would just talk. We would talk about how I was feeling that week. I had a lot of fear about getting over that first birth and would say, "Okay, that was *that* birth. This is going to be *this* birth, no matter how it turns out, whether it's a C-section or I have interventions. Whatever happens, I've got to be okay with it and honor it for that, for what it is, for the process it's going to be."

Jessica was wonderful. She would say, "Stop. Let's talk about how it's going to be okay no matter how it turns out. You're going to do great. You're going to give birth to a beautiful baby, a healthy baby. That is the goal. It's not about whether you have intervention or not." She talked about what the ideal birth looked like. And the more we talked, the more real it seemed. The more it felt like, "Yeah, I can do this." We did some relaxation techniques and visualization, and I practiced being really patient with myself and allowing myself to let go of feeling negative about Caroline's birth, acknowledging that all birth is a powerful, positive event.

I felt prepared for this birth, different than I felt the first time. This time I felt so centered and so at peace with whatever was going to come my way. I got to a point that even if it went down the same way that Caroline's went down, it was going to be different. I had had a baby before, so this wasn't foreign territory, and I had a support system. I had Jessica. I felt reinforced and like I was going in there with my guns loaded. So I felt very much at peace. I felt very tranquil.

Chloé was eight days overdue, but Caroline had been too, so I knew that due dates were irrelevant. I was ready Friday, December 19th when I woke up in the morning. I felt no contractions, not even Braxton Hicks contractions, but I had lost my mucus plug, so there were indications. The contractions I had that day were irregular. Some were an hour apart. Then at about one o'clock in the afternoon, they were about thirty minutes apart. They weren't at all painful. They were just these little bleeps. I thought, "Okay, my body is just getting ready."

I was still very laid back, not really thinking about it. Peter came home from work early, sick with the flu. He and Caroline napped, but I couldn't. I had energy, a *buzz*, which was very unusual because I'd been napping all throughout this pregnancy. My body knew something was happening, but I didn't. I took a walk around the neighborhood. It was drilled into my brain that if you're not dilated, if the contractions are not coming right on top of each other, they don't really mean anything. I thought, Maybe I'll have this baby in a couple of days.

We went to Peter's parents' house for dinner that night for distraction, to get us all out of the house. Peter was not feeling well, and we wanted to get Caroline over to see her grandparents. I wasn't having many contractions then; they had subsided. We had a nice evening. I think I even had some wine. We came home around nine thirty, and I lay down with Caroline to put her to bed. I had a killer contraction while I was lying down with her. I thought, "Okay, that was a *real* contraction."

Caroline fell asleep and I thanked God that she went to sleep before anything major kicked in. Then another contraction came about five or ten minutes later, and they kept coming. I looked at Peter lying in bed and I said, "Babe, I need you. You can't be sick right now. I'm sorry you're sick, but you cannot be sick *right now*." He got right up out of bed, put on his shirt, splashed his face with water, and said, "Okay." He rallied for me, which was great. I went to the other side of the bed, had a killer contraction, and my water broke.

We called Jessica during some of the early contractions, thinking she might want to sleep on the couch that night and that we might watch a few movies together because this was just the beginning. I thought I might go to the hospital Saturday morning around nine or ten o'clock. So when my water broke, we knew Jessica was on her way. By now the contractions were two to three minutes apart. Peter said, "I'd better call Mom and Dad," because they were going to come over and stay with Caroline. I was imagining everybody just sitting around wondering what we had all rallied for, because with Caroline it was so long.

I was squatting, hanging on to the side of the sink. That was great, and squatting was the best position for me during this birth. I was squatting on anything I could get my hands on. In between contractions, I had that blissful feeling of nothing going on. I would have this killer contraction, make guttural sounds like a monster, and then continue my conversation. "Well, anyway, like I was saying. . ." It was awesome. I didn't have that experience with Caroline. I worked myself up and had too much tension, so the time between contractions was not that blissful. But I was so aware of the in-between time with Chloé. It was just like skipping a beat. I would walk around the house lighting candles, have a contraction, and then put on some music. It was wonderful. The whole time I was thinking that this was just the beginning. The contractions were hard, but I was getting through them. Peter's mom, his dad, and Jessica arrived around ten thirty that night.

I had been reading some Bradley books about facial expressions in stages of labor. If you're chit-chatty you're not really there yet. Then you get a serious expression. Later, you get a *"Don't mess with me expression.*

JESSICA: I walked in the house and she was leaning over, hands on her knees, looking straight at me with her hair hanging in her face, totally serious. I said, "Something has happened since I talked to you on the phone." And she said, "Oh, I can't be ready. I don't have the serious expression." "You *have* the serious expression," I assured her.

PAMELA: Jessica watched me for a couple of contractions, and after the second contraction I did that same look where I was blowing the hair out of my face and squatting, looking at her, and I said, "We'd better go."

So we tried. But we couldn't find the keys to the car.

PETER: I'm Mr. Organized. Everything was packed. We were all set. But this took me by surprise. I don't know what we were thinking, but we thought we would have more time. So they all went outside and got into the car. I couldn't find the car keys. I finally went to my father and said, "You have to give me the keys to your car." So I had to go out and break the news to her—as she's going through a contraction—that she has to go from one car to the other. She was looking at me like. . .

PAMELA: I wasn't going to get out of that car. I was not going to. I just stayed there. But I did move to the back seat of the other car once I realized I wasn't going to have the baby for a while. While we drove, Jessica was applying pressure to my back, which was wonderful. I don't know how I could have made the ride there without somebody applying the pressure, because it was so essential. It gave me relief and it grounded me. We got to Kaiser at about eleven o'clock.

Now I felt the urge to push. It was intense. I felt that I needed to get my legs up around my ears and start pushing. I never had that with Caroline's birth. I just felt like I needed to do something more than what I was doing. So they tried to check me in at Kaiser. All I could hear was *blah, blah, blah.* I was just trying to find a room. I remember zigzagging around the halls like I was going to admit myself. I was just going to put myself in a room. Peter was downstairs parking the car, and Jessica was this wonderful guardian angel, directing me, and speaking coherently to the staff.

They changed my clothes. I knew I did not want a fetal monitor. I did not want the God-awful girdle on me. But I had to do it once. I think they did it once just to see that everything was copasetic. It was, so we took it right off. The nurse I had was wonderful, really sweet and supportive, but when she left the room, she left the room. I needed somebody to get that thing off me and to say, "It's okay, you don't need to have that on. You just need to do what feels right for you." And that is what Jessica kept saying over and over again. "Do what you need to do. If you feel like you need to push right now, push."

It was probably at that point that I was asking for an epidural, but they were so busy just trying to figure out where I was in the whole process. They examined me and I was dilated six centimeters. An hour later it was eight.

I was asking for pain relief. I had wanted to do it without drugs, but Jessica checked in with me in between contractions. She made eye contact and asked if I was sure I wanted the pain relievers. I started to trip all over myself apologizing because I was letting myself and Jessica down, but she came right back with "You've got to do what you've got to do." That gave me back my power. This was my decision. This was my body. This was my birth. That understanding was a drug for me. That was all I needed to make the switch. "Oh, thank you, you're right. Give me the Nubain!" Making that decision was never an issue after that.

After about half an hour I did get some Nubain and that was all I needed. It was just enough to keep me from going over the edge with the contractions. I had a small recovery period after each contraction subsided, but just for a nanosecond. I didn't have time for an epidural, and I don't think I would have wanted one anyway. I just needed to take the edge off. I felt like I could do it.

I have a sweet memory of this birth. It was during one of the contractions at the hospital. Jessica was on one side of me and Peter was on the other. At one point Peter and I put our heads together, and I had the most tender sort of "Oh, we're doing this together" feeling. It was a connection. It was wonderful, so sweet and special. I wanted the father of this child to be a part of it. I hope I never forget that because that was really, really tender and sweet.

Then the birth moved with lightning speed. I remember saying to the nurse at twelve thirty, between contractions, "Gee, when do you think this baby's going to come?" I was thinking about six o'clock in the morning, and she said, "This baby is going to be here by one o'clock this morning." I looked at the clock and thought, "Poor thing, she doesn't know what she's talking about. Where'd she go to nursing school?"

I said I had to push, and probably at that point they were telling me not to. The doctor hadn't come yet to examine me, and I'm sure they were afraid of tearing and all kinds of stuff like that. But the urge to push was so strong. Again, Jessica said, "If you need to push, you push." And I listened to her. I trusted her, so I did push and it felt great and it felt right. It felt like I was working with my body. I don't think I could have stopped pushing—it was too strong, too there, and it felt too right. So I just kept pushing.

The doctor came in and sat down, and said, "Okay, we're ready. Let's go, we're doing this." She was wearing one of those big high-tech masks, and I thought, "Wow, Darth Vader is delivering my baby." She was very calm. The lights were low. It was such a different birth. I remember only the last two pushes really burned and hurt. I kept saying, "No, I can't do this." You know, the typical things you say. "I can't do this. Forget about it."

Then Dr. B was saying, "Pamela, touch your baby's head." She was trying to get me to lean forward and touch. I knew what she was trying to do and I wasn't going to. So I said, "No, no, no. I can't do it." And she said, "Yes, you can." And she said it so emphatically, and Jessica and Peter were saying, "Yes, you can. It's there. Look at your baby's head." At that point I was delirious. But I heard Jessica. I heard Dr. B, and I saw Chloé's head reflected in her mask.

Behind Dr. B was the bathroom, and in the shower door I could see everything. I saw a mirror image of what was going on. I saw my legs. And I saw this body coming out. It was almost like an out of body experience. I was watching this birth, and it was like all the videos I had seen, but it was me. The environment was so mellow. I did that last push and there was that relief, that slippery, wonderful relief. I felt the three stages: head, shoulders, and the whole twist of the body coming out. I was aware of all of it. I felt the head come out and the burning was gone, but there was still an incredible amount of pressure during that brief rest. I think I said, "We don't even know if it's a boy or a girl!" Dr. B said, "I'll tell you. Don't worry." Right at one o'clock in the morning, it was a girl. Seven pounds, ten ounces, twenty-one and a half inches long. Long and lean. She came right up onto my tummy and to my breast. She was mad, mad, mad, and she must have screamed for forty-five minutes.

PETER: I was looking at the head, remembering. What I was doing the whole time was remembering Caroline's birth. I was thinking, "Okay, where are we, in what stage?" It was going so fast that my head was spinning. I was battling this flu, not even feeling that much any more, but I was thinking, "My God, everything is going so fast. Okay. She pushed. Okay, there's the head. Okay, a little more," and all of a sudden they're holding this baby! I was thinking, "When did that happen?" I can't even rewind it. I don't even know what happened in between. Even when she came out, I didn't think about whether she was a boy or a girl. I was just thinking, "Wow, look at our baby. Our baby is out." I got to cut the umbilical cord this time too, which was completely different from Caroline. Here was Pamela, walking around ten minutes after giving birth, and our baby screaming, and we're going, "Wow, this is incredible." Caroline was so quiet, not a peep. Everything about it all was a night-and-day experience.

PAMELA: The placenta was easy—one push. I had the same sense of relief when it was delivered, but none of the pain or awareness of it coming out. It was just another step closer toward the whole cycle being completed. When the placenta was delivered, I really relaxed.

Chloé didn't nurse right away. She was very upset and had just gone through an obviously unbelievable journey, so I forgave her that and let her scream her lungs out. I guess I hadn't fully forgiven myself for asking for Nubain, and I said to the nurse, "What effect would Nubain have on her? What should I look for?" and she said, "Respiratory problems." There was Chloé, screaming a blue streak, obviously having no trouble breathing, and it was just perfect.

Again, it was another validation. I had made the right decision for myself and for my baby. They did what they needed to do with her after I tried to nurse, and we looked at her and bonded with her, even though she was so mad. And I was in the bathroom chatting with the nurse ten minutes after I had the baby. I felt so empowered. I felt like I could just get right up and walk right out of that hospital. Take my baby, thank them for the bed, and just go. I didn't need to be there at all. Jessica thinks that losing the keys was a sign from God that we should have had a homebirth, and I almost believe that.

When Caroline and Chloé grow up, I will tell them to have support when they go through a birth—an outside source of support, not a mother-in-law, sister-in-law, aunt, or cousin. It's nice to have a third party around because that keeps everything in perspective. It keeps everything going and keeps everybody on a level field. The second birth wouldn't have been as wonderful an experience without Jessica. Even though it was a great birth and everything was beautiful and we came out of it empowered and feeling fantastic, there might still have been complications. It was just nice to have that extra person there knowing what's going on, giving us advice. You have an outside force if it does get complicated.

You have to create a community. The hospitals have their agenda. Other people have their agendas. But it has to be the Mom's and Dad's agenda, and ultimately, the Mom's agenda that's most important. The family needs to form a supportive community around them.

A lot of women, and I was one of them, put a lot of faith in the medical establishment and in the doctors and the nurses. I thought I would be safe and cared for at the hospital. I don't want to make it sound like an evil, awful place, but it wasn't at all what I thought it was.

There is a point where you have too much information, and that's what happened to us with the first one. There's a point when you have to go with your instincts. You cannot base your experience on a textbook or on what another person says. They very well might know what they're doing but it's not right for you at that time. So a person has to go with her instincts and if she feels it's right, she has to be strong enough to say, "This is what I want. This is the way I want it to be."

JESSICA: I saw it all coming from within you. It was so beautiful to watch you during the times we met beforehand. The reason this birth was so great wasn't because you had a doula. It was because you found that peace inside.

PAMELA: I kept repeating an affirmation called "Chant for Transition." It had some phrases that just clicked for me, like, "The intensity brings the baby. . . The baby's coming. . . This is bringing your baby." Well of course it is, but you don't think of that when you're in labor because it really hurts. You're thinking, "What am I doing this for?" So to have Peter and Jessica to say that affirmation to me made all the difference and I'd say, "Okay, I am opening a door and this is a passage. This is not someone torturing me. This is bringing somebody into the world."

PETER: As soon as you try to organize it, it's not going to work. Whatever you organize, it's not going to work that way anyway. Just be there for her and do what she wishes because that is the only thing you're there for. That is it—to be supportive to the Mom—because you can have all the organizational skills in the world and it doesn't matter. The keys are still lost. It just doesn't matter.

BABY WANTS OUT!

SUELI AND MARCUS

Although she delivered in a hospital, Sueli needed none of the medical interventions available there. She was overjoyed that her labor and delivery were managed quite well by Mother Nature.

Sueli is from Brazil; she met and married Frank after he saw her dancing the samba one night. Sueli, her sisters, and her cousins were all born at home in Brazil with the help of a midwife. Her culture accepted birth as a natural, normal process, certainly not anything a hospital needed to manage. Sueli seems to travel through life as if she were floating on a gently flowing stream, enjoying the ride, accepting whatever comes along with great delight. Her positive attitude throughout her pregnancy, labor, and delivery is apparent in her story. Perhaps this positive attitude is because she comes from a different culture; perhaps it's because she comes from a large family—a family that gave her a way of seeing birth as a normal part of life. Sueli saw her pregnancy as "making magic happen" and quickly countered any fears by calling her sisters and mother on the phone and listening to their calm words.

What I will never forget about Sueli were her cries as each pushing contraction started. She would call out, "Baby wants *out!*" and commence pushing with all her might. Marcus weighed eight pounds, one ounce when he was born, and Sueli truly appreciated the work the baby did during her labor to help the birth process.

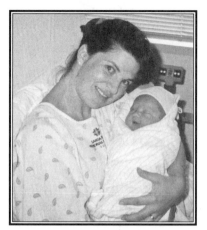

Sueli and Marcus

SUELI: I am Sueli, and this is the story of the birth of Marcus. He was born on July 6, 1996—a summer baby.

My pregnancy went very smoothly. I had a wonderful pregnancy. I felt like I was living in a special little world and that I was making magic and everything around me was just perfect. We never had a difficult situation during the entire pregnancy. I was really lucky to have it go so well. It may have been because we had planned it. We were sure we wanted a baby, were prepared, and knew this was the right time. We decided that we wanted to do it now, and it happened really easily because I got pregnant on the first try. I had a lot of support from everyone around me. I worked at a school, and lots of teachers and wonderful people were always talking about it and sharing this and that. They would tell their stories, and I was always telling them how I felt. Most of the stories were good.

My mom had six babies. I'm the fourth, and I don't think labor was ever difficult for her. Having babies in my family was an easy thing to do, just a natural thing. I was very healthy, and I was working and exercising at work, walking around and just being very busy all the time. I was feeling my best, making my little miracle.

Then we started the childbirth preparation classes. That scared me because they told me about Cesarean births, difficult births, and sixteen-hour labors, and I thought, "Oh my gosh!" I was concerned. So I called home and I asked, "Mom, do you remember how your labor went?" And she said, "Oh, it was so long ago!" She had all of us at home with a midwife because that is what they did at the time. There was no going to the hospital or worrying about C-sections or anything. It was always done at home, very informally.

She said that when she was little, her older sisters would come to her mother's house to have their babies. She remembers there would be some people running around and getting busy and then they would lock the door of the bedroom. A few moments later they had a baby, then they'd play with the baby, and that was it. It was such a natural thing.

Then I asked my sisters about their labor. One said, "The first went well and the second time I had a C-section, but it was fine." And the same story from another sister, "It only took me a couple of hours." And so I relaxed a little.

I went to the books and read everything. I read some articles that I thought had good suggestions and good advice. I went back and read those articles over and over.

One hot Friday night, I had a big dinner and then we tried to watch a movie. It was two weeks before I was due; I wasn't expecting anything to happen. But after dinner, we tried to watch this movie and I just couldn't get comfortable. Any position on the couch wouldn't do, and I was getting very irritated and said, "Gosh I feel like my dinner is stuck here, and I'm not comfortable."

I tried to lie down and used two pillows, but nothing helped. I went upstairs and said to Frank, "I'm going to take a shower. By the way, why don't

Childbirth classes are good for general information about the process and what to expect, but be careful to avoid horror stories and negative expectations. Remember: Having babies naturally has been a successful process and happy occasion for many centuries.

you just go ahead and take me to the hospital? *I'm ready.* I'm *tired* of this." I had stopped working and was just waiting for the baby to come. This was my summer thing; I had nothing planned but having a baby. I'd been waiting for two weeks at home. I couldn't go to the mall anymore or go shopping or enjoy anything because I was very heavy and my feet would get tired and my back would hurt. So I couldn't enjoy the summer.

I went and had a shower to relax a little. I took a cold shower because it was hot. Then, that was it. I went to bed and at four o'clock my water broke and woke me up. I thought, "Whoooaaaaa! Warm water!" And I was so happy, you wouldn't believe it. I was laughing and said, "We're having a baby. We're going to come home with a baby today!" There we were, smelling the water and laughing. "They said it would smell like baby pee, but it doesn't!"

We managed to go back to bed. We decided to rest because if we had fourteen hours ahead of us, we wanted to save our energy. We really were planning to go back to sleep but of course, neither of us could sleep at that point. There we were in bed for about an hour, just talking about it, "Ah, so that's why I was so irritated last night and couldn't get comfortable."

And then Frank said, "Don't we have to go to the hospital? In the class they said if the water breaks, you have to go to the hospital."

"Yeah but that's for you, for the father who doesn't know what to do. We have a long time to wait. Why go to the hospital right now?" I knew it would be at least six or seven hours.

So we decided to relax and stay home. That was my plan, to stay home until I was ready to go. By five thirty, we had to get out of bed and Frank said, "What would you like for breakfast? I'll cook you up some breakfast." We had oatmeal and then called Dr. Stacey at about six o'clock. The contractions had started by then, but we were still comfortable being at home. I called my friend Karen at about eight o'clock and told her, "Hey guess what, I'm in labor!" I was totally happy—not nervous at all—relaxed because everything was going really well just like the books described it.

I was basically by myself. Frank was packing; he was getting ready. He had to put the car seat in the car, grab all the stuff to do back massages if it was a back labor, and prepare the Lamaze bag. So I was kind of on my own at home. And that was good because Frank is really great, but sometimes he's too much.

Dr. Stacey told me to call whenever I was ready, when I couldn't handle it at home anymore. By nine o'clock, the pain was really intense, and I was having really scary contractions. So, I decided, "I want to go to the hospital so that I can have the drugs if I need them." I knew that I had to be about four or five centimeters.

I don't know if I can describe the pain. I always thought this about it: The baby wants to come out. I had a lot of Braxton Hicks contractions throughout the pregnancy, and these felt the same. These contractions were just like my body getting ready to deliver the baby. They were okay. I was breathing and relaxing, especially relaxing my lower back. I would sometimes get on the door frame and press against it, and the

Most women know when they want to be at the hospital, when they no longer want to be at home with their contractions. By that time, the adrenaline that comes with a change in environment is not enough to stop labor and they are less likely to get unnecessary interventions.

contractions would come and I could handle them. But it wasn't a weird pain or even a normal pain. It's different, but I just don't know how to describe it.

I did lose control when I threw up. I kind of got scared and I lost control right there. That's when I said, "All right, we really need to go to the hospital." Because then the pain was really strong and I thought I may need help. I think at that point it did overwhelm me a little. We were open for whatever we needed. We did not want to be stuck with "We don't want drugs," and then, well, die, or have a terrible labor. We wanted to do whatever was necessary to have a nice labor, so drugs were an option.

Sueli was not rigid in any way about her labor. Her flexibility helped her open up and have a smooth labor.

We got to the hospital and Frank dropped me off right in front and went to park. Then he came back, and we walked into the hospital. I remember we were in the elevator, I was having contractions, and there were about five people staring at me. I was trying not to show that I was in labor. I was feeling great, totally under control again. Then I walked to the nurse's station at the very end of the hall and said, "I'm in labor." They looked at me and said, "Are you sure?" I'll never forget that. "Of course I'm sure; I've been in labor since five thirty this morning!" And it was almost ten.

They were expecting me because Stacey had called, but they were kind of busy. So, a nurse came in and said, "Okay, now lie down and we'll get the monitor to see how the baby's doing."

I said, "I don't know, I think I need to go to the bathroom," but then I couldn't move. I just could not move. I managed to walk towards the bed but by then she had left again. When she came back, I was still standing there and I said, "I can't move. I need help." I was really ready.

It was just the nurse, Frank, and me. So I was still kind of on my own. I did get onto the bed with some help, but I was doing my thing and I knew everything was okay. I had the nurse intervening every now and then and checking on me. And of course, when she first checked, I was fully dilated. She said, "Oh my gosh, you're ready to push and we're not ready for you! But whenever you feel like pushing you can start."

It was funny because there I was ready, and again I was so thrilled that I didn't have to go through five centimeters. . . seven centimeters. . . nine centimeters... You know. I was just ready. It felt like it was almost over, and that was so positive because I didn't have to worry anymore. Great, we don't have to think about massages or walking around the halls! Forget it, it's almost done. That was really great. I felt so good. Yes! Yes! It was worth being home and relaxing, taking showers, and just breathing, like we learned in class. I felt the nurses' panic, but it didn't really bother me. They were rushing, but I was so happy. Hey, I'm almost done here. I felt like I was at home. I was relaxed since they were there, and I had the assistance I needed, and I didn't need drugs at all because I was relaxed and dilated.

I didn't really know how to push. I was thinking that there really was no way at home that we could have practiced that like we did with the relaxing techniques, because I couldn't really push before. I wouldn't take the chance. And the first few times I tried to push, I really didn't know how and I wasn't doing a good job. But I think when Stacey started directing me, she would say, "Do you feel here? Then that's where you have to push," that helped me. And the nurse was also very good. She was speaking to me very softly. I remember her by my right ear and she would say, "Okay now, next time it comes, push hard and breathe and relax and then let's get this baby out." She was really good. I liked the way she behaved during the labor. She was just barely there, so I was again in total control and I had her there to help me and my doctor was there. But nobody pushed me. I was just doing my thing.

It took me two hours to get the baby out.

When the baby got close to the outside, it hurt. I was prepared for that because I had read about it, and in class they kind of prepared you for it. They were always saying how it's going to burn and you have to push through it. Dr. Stacey told me the same thing too, during labor. And so I was expecting that pain to come because that meant it was almost over. I was kind of looking forward to it. At that point I really wanted the baby out and was always saying, during every contraction, "*Baby wants ooooooouuuuuut*" and then I would start screaming and pushing. I remember when the head came through and Frank said, "Oh, I can see this much of the head . . ." I do remember the body going through. I will never forget that, like the baby was slipping through—just so wonderful.

Then I felt that weight on my stomach. I was very tired at that point. I think I had my eyes closed because I had pushed so

Looking forward to pushing your baby with excited anticipation makes it easier to accept and push through the pain.

hard. I looked and said, "Oh, my God, this is my baby! "It took about ten or twelve seconds, and then Frank asked, "Well, what is it?" So I looked and said, "It's a boy!" It was great. He was so big and heavy, and that's what I felt on my stomach.

He didn't cry right away and I was a little concerned, but I had that positive, wishing feeling that it would be fine. Of course, he was fine. I remember saying, "Come on baby, now you have to cry." I think he was a little too tired, but he cried later!

I remembered the placenta had to come, and I heard Stacey say, "Okay, push again," and then I pushed and it was kind of weird. It hurt.

And then I was done.

Sometime in the next hour, the baby tried to nurse. I couldn't do it right away. I think we knew that he would be perfectly awake and aware, and we waited for that. We nursed for the first time when it was just the three of us in the room. He was clean, he was ready, and then we did it.

I was in the hospital for about twenty-four hours. I was ready to come home; I missed my bed and my house. But when I got home, I wished that I had stayed a little longer because I was kind of afraid to be by myself with the baby. Frank was there, but we didn't have any experience with babies. My family is in Brazil, and his family was not really ready to be there with us at that point.

It's a good idea to arrange for a friend or family member to be there when you first take your baby home. That way you can sleep and bond and get breastfeeding going properly while someone you trust supports the workings of the household.

When I tell my story to Marcus and his wife, I will say that my birth story is a positive story. Your body knows how to do the whole thing. Don't fight it. You just need to be there and let it happen.

❋

I simply *love* Sueli's advice because it doesn't get any simpler, sweeter, or truer. So I repeat for her: You just need to be there and let it happen.

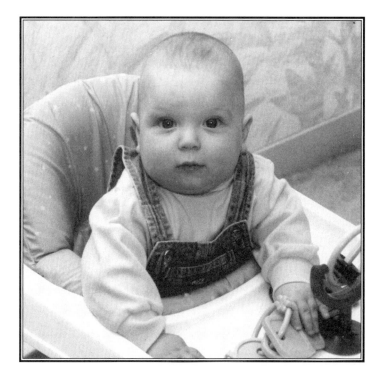

Marcus Okun

As Simple as It Gets

Jennifer and Akayla

Jennifer works for a pharmaceutical company, and her husband Greg is a carpenter with his own business. Akayla was their first child.

It is important to remember that the majority of births are uncomplicated. They are always full of drama, but most of the time babies are born safely with no need for techno-medical heroics. And Jennifer's birth story is about as simple as it gets. She prepared by taking prenatal classes, avoiding scary stories, and hanging on to anything positive that she heard. Jennifer knows herself well, knows that she has a chronic anxiety disorder, and knows the tools she can use to manage that anxiety without medication. She works out at a gym on a regular basis. Yes, she enjoys it, but more importantly this is the way she stays calm. Regular cardiovascular workouts help keep the panic attacks away, so even during the pregnancy, she pushed herself at the gym several times a week. These invaluable tools stood her in good stead during Akayla's birthing.

With her ability to focus on a goal, her physical conditioning, and no medical problems to increase her risks, Jennifer was a perfect candidate for a midwifery-model birth. She imagined she was doing bench press reps when she was in transition and that allowed her to accept the intensity of the moment, knowing that it would not last forever.

Jennifer went into this birth with no set expectations. Her baby's birth could have easily happened at home with a midwife, but she and Greg chose the reassurance of a hospital setting, so they integrated Jennifer's focused but uncomplicated approach with the supportive environment of the hospital. So simple.

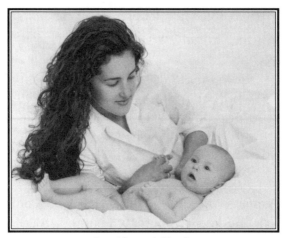

Jennifer and Akayla

JENNIFER: When I arrived at the hospital, I kept thinking, "Well, soon we'll have a baby." Whatever that means. During the whole birthing process I just kind of disconnected myself from the whole thing. I just kept thinking of the following day. How can you conceptualize it if you've never been through it? You've seen all these other things. You've heard everybody's story, but now it's finally happening to you. I went to class, I did not read all the scary books, and I hung onto the positive stories.

I went in for my checkup at a week past due, and they wanted to break my water. I had been walking around for two weeks at three centimeters. It was a full moon the night before and I had mild contractions the whole night, about ten minutes apart and lasting for about forty-five seconds. They were super-duper mild. When I got up to relax with it, it stopped. Then I went to the hospital, my doctor broke the water, and we did nipple stimulation and a lot of walking.

Allowing the provider to rupture the membranes is a relatively natural way of inducing labor without the side effects of medication. But breaking the water should not be done without careful consideration because once the membranes are ruptured, the baby must be born within twenty-four hours or the chance of infection becomes a concern.

About three hours later, the contractions started to happen regularly—first about eight minutes apart and then three minutes apart. I didn't know what was going on so I just kept walking and walking. I got tired and bored with walking. Greg walked with me the whole time, and about the time the contractions got regular and stronger, my family arrived. So I had my mother and my father and my cousins following me around at times. Then they would go sit down. I was wondering, "Now what? What else is going to happen?"

Finally I started to get some really yucky contractions. What was amazing is that I thought the contractions were going to be shooting pains. But it felt like when you're having diarrhea or painful menstrual cramps. The great thing about it was that they would only last for so long and then I would get a little break. I felt like I was walking around forever and I kept asking the nurse, "When is it going to happen? I don't want to do anything that is going to slow this process down. What can I do?" She offered to give me some kind of shot of something to take the edge off, to make me more comfortable. She said it was like having two margaritas. So I said okay and it did take the edge off. It made me kind of sleepy and made me feel kind of funny. I was laughing, we were walking around, and then about half an hour later it wore off.

Nurses may suggest pain medication because that is what they have to offer. It doesn't mean you have to accept it and it doesn't mean that it will help your labor be more effective. Jennifer didn't really need this medicine, but she decided to give it a try.

I was being checked every half-hour and was at about five centimeters when I started throwing up. I started to get really frustrated with the whole thing. Nothing was funny anymore. I was over trying to be cool. I asked my whole family to leave and then only Greg was in there. I was sitting in the rocking chair and asked the nurse, "What can I do? I'm through with this now. I'm frustrated." I was trying to be polite to her saying, "I know this is your job and everything but I just want to hold this together. What can I do?" She just said, "Keep relaxing." I couldn't tell if I was having a contraction or if I was just making it up. One contraction would be over and then another would start to come and I remember bending over and wondering, "Okay is this one or not?" Greg would come over and say, "Breathe," and that would help me disassociate myself from the experience. I would think about what I was going to do tomorrow. I would fantasize about what the next day would be like.

It didn't hurt. It felt like when I was sitting on the toilet with diarrhea and terrible cramps, and I thought, "Oh my God, when is this going to end?" And to me that's discomfort, not pain. So I guess it's just my definition.

When I was at eight centimeters I said, "I don't think I'm going to make it. I'm sick, I'm uncomfortable. What can I do to speed it up? I want to do anything to speed it up. I don't think I can make it. Is it time now? Can I have something for pain?" The nurse looked at me and said, "Jennifer, when things are falling apart is when they finally come together. I'll be back in half an hour and I'm going to bring you some good news."

Now they were three minutes apart and I thought they had to be on top of each other for you to have the baby. She gave me another shot and it didn't help me relax, it just made me tired. It made me groggy and I didn't like it. Every time a contraction would come I'd say, "Okay here comes another one," and Greg didn't know what to do. I'd have a contraction and I'd tell him to start rubbing my back. Then I'd say, "No it's not my back! Stop, stop, stop!" It would radiate from the middle of my back down my lower back to the front lower abdomen.

He'd say, "I don't know what to do!" and I'd say, "Rub my arms, squeeze my arms." I didn't really yell and scream at him, so it got to the point that we were doing hand signals. I was doing thumbs up for "okay" and was shaking my hand for "no." One of the things they taught me in the birthing class was about tensing up another part of your body. So I would do that, I would tense up my arms and focus on that. Grip, grip, grip my hand. At this point Greg had to take his wedding ring off because it was cutting the circulation off in his hand.

That half-hour was awful. Absolutely horrible. I hated it. I was walking and sitting and saying to myself, "Why do people do this? Why do people want to come back and do this?" I was dead serious. I said, "I don't really care to do this ever again. I don't enjoy it. I'm very uncomfortable. I'm pissed off." For me it didn't hurt. It made me feel like punching something or somebody.

When I am in pain, I always get really angry. It's just what I do. I squeezed Greg's hand really tight and looked over the horizon. I had a spot on the hill out the window that I could see and I would concentrate on that and breathe. And I'd count, and in forty-five seconds, it was over. It was like a rep when I work out at the gym, when I do those last two reps and it's painful and then it's over. And then I get to rest. I was imagining that I was exercising, working out, doing a bench press.

When my nurse came back after a half an hour, she said there was just a little cervix left and we could try pushing a little bit. She called the doctor and had me start pushing. I didn't know that when you call the doctor, that means things are going to start happening! Pushing felt tight and hard, just like everybody described. Pressure. Okay, I do need to say this: Nothing felt like people had described it because I did not know what to expect. There was pressure, but it wasn't painful and I just didn't get it. It was difficult because I didn't know how hard I was pushing. They told me the position I was supposed to be in with my knees up by my throat, one person on one side and Greg on the other. And I was supposed to push like I was taking the biggest dump of my life. I'm trying to push as hard as I can and the doctor is telling me, "Every millimeter counts. You have to keep your legs all the way up to your chest and push as hard as you can."

When women think they've reached their absolute limit, they are often in transition and close to completely dilated. It helps to have someone remind you of this when you think you can't do it anymore.

Being overwhelmed can feel like anger, and that kind of energy can be focused. But don't let your nurse or coach say, "That's right! Get angry! Get that baby out!" Try to birth your baby with strength, but not with rage.

Remember that there are many different positions for pushing and you should get to choose which one works best for you. It can also help to have your provider guide you into effective pushes so you know that your efforts are working.

Well, this was none of the stuff they do in movies! No fancy coaching, just, "Take a deep breath and go for it!" So now Greg has one arm over my knee, the other arm behind my neck and he's squeezing me together and I'm pushing. The thing that got me through my twenty minutes of pushing was that I imagined Greg and myself working out, lifting weights. Every time I pushed, I imagined lifting something *really* super heavy, and I did this horrible grunting. Deep breath, push, and she's telling me there is something happening down there, but I couldn't feel anything. I just felt numb with a lot of pressure. My throat was getting very dry and hoarse from the grunting.

After ten minutes of this, it seemed like it had been going on forever and I was thinking, "They're going to want to do a C-section! I know it. I've already been through all this and now they're going to do a C-section." It was really making me angry. I couldn't tell if I was having a contraction. It was just tons of pressure. If it weren't for Greg telling me to breathe and focus, I would have flown off the table. The funny thing is, I kept complaining, "I'm not strong. I'm a weakling!" and he would say, "The hell you're not! You're strong!" I had my arm around his arm pushing back against his pulling on me. Then, all of a sudden, I looked in the mirror and I could see the head. That was the weirdest, most surreal experience of my life. The whole head was popping out.

The whole time I was pregnant I was thinking, "Yes, I'm pregnant, but what does that really mean? Is there really a little person in there?" The head came out and I thought, "That little round head came out, now those big wide shoulders have to come out."

The doctor laid her right on my chest and belly. She had her little arm poking straight out at me, with her little head lying on it looking right at me. She had a perfectly round head. She was almost pink. We all looked and realized she was a girl. I didn't cry. Greg didn't cry. We were a bit teary eyed, but it was very surreal. She took the biggest poop and got that black tar all over everybody.

The doctor pressed on my stomach and all this stuff came out and then another push and the placenta came out. I sat up and said, "I want to see it." So she told me all about it. It was amazing.

Seeing the top of your baby's head peeking out can be incredibly motivational and can make the whole process suddenly real. Don't be afraid to look, or even to reach down and touch your baby for the first time.

During the whole pushing thing you don't care about a thing. Just get it out. I kept thinking that I did not go through all this to have somebody not healthy come out. It was really odd thinking afterwards, "Now I have this full human." I'm an intelligent, breathing, caring person. I knew this was going to happen, but now that it had happened, now what? My family came in and they all said, "Isn't it all wonderful?" I was just very content with the whole thing—having her, looking at her, seeing her, and holding her.

I wasn't afraid of childbirth at all. And that doesn't make an ounce of sense at all. It's just something that you have to tough out. I didn't take more pain medicine because I knew I would still be uncomfortable and after the whole thing was over, I'd be hung over. I'd think that tomorrow is going to be a new day and it's going to be better and I won't be feeling like this anymore. I'd just think of the horizon and what lay ahead, and I didn't dwell on what was going on at the moment.

I wasn't excited about it. I was just really indifferent to the whole experience. I thought that would be really painful, so I just grunted as hard as I could and the whole thing just popped right out. I felt her entire body come out and it was the neatest

Jennifer avoided all negative stories. Neither did she fantasize about creating a beautiful birth. She decided to keep it simple, be practical, and do whatever it took at the time to get her baby out.

feeling, like nothing I'd ever felt. It was such a relief, such an "Ahhhhhh…." Almost like exhaling. I felt great afterwards. It was so strange.

The whole birthing process was very surreal, a completely altered state of consciousness. When I sum up the whole labor and birthing process, it was really an hour and a half of uncomfortable stuff. It was easy. On the other hand, it was the hardest thing I've ever done. It just wasn't what I expected. I expected to be totally exhausted and thought it would be very painful. While I was in the middle of it I kept thinking, "This is not something I ever want to do again. If I do do it, I hope I forget about it like everybody says. Maybe I will." The neat thing about it is that today, it has become a special experience. Now I see what everybody is talking about. You just don't really know what you're going to experience because everybody's experience is so unique.

It was the most wonderful, best, most fabulous thing that has happened in my entire life. I'm eating my words, but I'm looking forward to having another one!

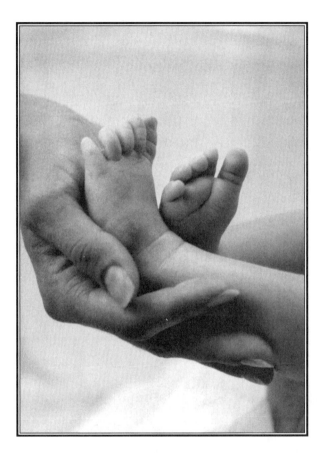

Sliding into Home

Serena and Sophie

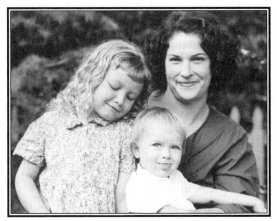

Serena, Bryna, and Sophie

I love this story. Serena's sense of humor never failed her. During the hardest part of her labor, while she was beside herself trying to get an epidural, she was still one of the most genuine and delightful women I had ever worked with. This birth is a good representation of all good births that are like thrilling roller coaster rides—a bit scary at the start, almost too intense in the midst of it all, and exhilarating at the successful end. Simply wonderful.

Labor did not start spontaneously for either of Serena's births, and this is a source of sadness for her. After she waited three weeks past her due date without going into labor, her first birthing was controlled with Pitocin, start to finish. Serena is a practical woman; she didn't dwell on her disappointment and hoped for the best the second time around. With the excited anticipation of every pregnant woman, she waited to go into labor spontaneously at the end of her second pregnancy. Nothing happened. Ten days past her due date, we agreed to start the induction. None of us was willing to wait a possible three full weeks again. Serena was calm and sure about being induced. She did not expect her second labor to be much different than the first one, but she was in for a big surprise. She had no idea that her body could kick in with its own labor-inducing chemicals. She was about to find out that the combination of Pitocin and natural hormones can bring on a labor that is overwhelmingly intense and productive.

I sent Serena to the hospital that evening so that the nurses could help us ripen her cervix. This involved putting some medicinal gel up next to her cervix and letting it soften the tissue overnight in anticipation of opening up to ten centimeters the next day. Sometimes this ripening is enough to get labor going all by itself, but in Serena's case it didn't work. She needed Pitocin.

I came to the hospital the next morning to check Serena's cervix, to see if she still wanted Pitocin, and to check on the baby. She definitely wanted to get things going, so we started a bit of IV Pitocin and she quickly went into hard labor. I left her and her husband Eric to labor as a family for awhile. It wasn't long before I got a call that she was asking for an epidural, so I made my way back over to the hospital to see how she was doing and discuss the pain situation. Serena was adamant, and because Pitocin can cause harsh contractions, I certainly understood her need. The trouble was, it was Saturday and we only had one anesthesiologist available on the weekend. That doctor was tied up in a surgery for several more hours and we were going to have to wait. Hours passed. No one but her husband could stay in the room for very long because none of us had what she wanted: an epidural. It was getting harder and harder to keep her focused and more and more challenging to help her maintain her sense of humor.

I remembered a technique I had read about in one of my journals. Injecting sterile water just under the skin in two points on the lower back can give great relief to women with painful back labor. Serena was having back labor and this sounded like just the stopgap measure we needed. So she sat on the soft birthing ball while I gave her the injections. The technique did give her just enough relief to stay on top of the contractions. But an hour later, her labor pain was back in full force. The pain was making her irritable, and Serena would not let me check her cervix. She was laboring on that big ball and did not want to move, so we agreed that

I would check her when the anesthesiologist came in to do the epidural. We continued to monitor the baby's heart with a portable Doppler every so often to make sure the baby was doing well. But we had no idea how quickly Serena was progressing.

I waited outside her room so I could catch the anesthesiologist as soon as he came out of surgery, and although I was standing fifteen feet away, I almost missed this delivery. I looked up to see Eric barreling through the door with an expression on his face that could not be misinterpreted. Charging into the room, I grabbed a glove and slid across the floor to reach under Serena's squatting bottom. There was not a moment to spare. I caught Sophie's head, inches from the floor. The birthing ball rolled off into the corner as Serena plopped back into Eric's arms and down on the floor to receive her baby into her arms.

What made this particular birth integrative? Serena and I worked together throughout both her pregnancies, balancing her desire for natural childbirth with the need to help Mother Nature. With her first pregnancy, I could have pushed her to induce a week earlier than we did. The protocol in most hospitals is to wait no longer than forty-two weeks before delivering the baby. The risk of losing the baby goes up significantly two weeks after a due date, and we talked about this. But instead we chose to watch carefully, to closely monitor her baby and the placental support system, and to come to a decision together about the best time to induce.

Through that pregnancy and delivery, Serena and I created a relationship of trust and friendship. So when her second baby was late, I knew Serena would discuss her desires with me and that they would be realistic and appropriate. She knew the risks of waiting. She accepted those risks but was not impractical. She knew she had the final say and that allowed her to make a wise decision rather than react to protocols or someone else's attempts to control her birth. Had we followed the medical model during her labor, we would have kept her in bed, checked her cervix regularly, and kept the fetal monitors on her at all times. But Serena was doing well on that labor ball and didn't want to move. We were listening to the baby's heart frequently and knew she was doing fine. There was no real need to disturb Serena as long as the baby continued to do well. We stayed with her, gave her all the support we could, and used every possible alternative to an epidural. These are wonderful examples of integrative childbirth: helping Mother Nature by doing only what is necessary, maintaining a trusting communicative relationship, and making decisions collaboratively.

After this birth, the family gave me a catcher's mitt that still hangs on the wall of my office above the pictures of the babies I have delivered. I smile every time I see it and remember Serena's power, her practicality, her humor, and the epidural that didn't happen.

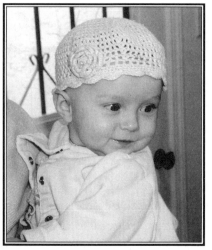

Sophie

SERENA: My first pregnancy with Bryna was calm and serene and I walked about an inch above the ground the whole time. And then Bryna was three weeks late. Each week that she was late I got more and more bummed. But I was never really scared about going into labor or having her. I just figured that labor would be no problem. When I was three weeks late and had to be induced, I was really disappointed that my body didn't kick in by itself, but the labor part of it, the pushing and all that stuff, was so instinctual that it was really easy. I figured that every cell of my body and every cell of every creature on the planet is told what it's supposed to do: procreate. I figured that, at some point, my cells would come together and figure it out and do it correctly. I really believed that. I didn't have any fear at all about that part.

Both girls were planned. This is how I knew it was time to get pregnant again: Every day when we would have to go to the store, we would pass a little carousel in front. I would say to Bryna, "After we do the grocery shopping, we'll ride on the carousel," and every day she would cry as we were going by. One day I said, "After we go grocery shopping, you can ride on that carousel." And she said, "Okay Momma, I'll wait." And then I said, "Oh, I can have another one." I knew I was ready because now I could reason with the first one. Bryna was three years and two months old when Sophie was born.

We decided to try getting pregnant in September. I think I probably got pregnant on September 1st because Sophie was born nine months later!

Ten days past my due date, there was no sign of my going into labor. I was so ready to have her and be a nursing mom, to be home and taking my kids to the park. I know Dr. Stacey sensed that. I was so ready to have our family of two kids, one on each arm, complete. So when I was ten days late, I remembered that Bryna was twenty-one days late and I never did go into labor. I thought, "I'm not going to wait twenty-one days again." I talked to Dr. Stacey, and we planned to induce this birth before I went much further.

We left Bryna with her godmother, and Eric and I went to have a nice dinner. Then we casually strolled over to the hospital hand in hand, lah dee dah dee dah. Even though I chose to be induced, I was definitely disappointed that I wasn't able to start up the whole birth process on my own.

We tried putting gel on my cervix, which is not necessarily fun. I mean there's no joy in it, but there's not much pain either. It's just one of those things you have to do. It's a little achy and not terribly painful, but it is a medical procedure, so there is some unpleasantness involved. My husband, not respecting at all that we might be in active labor, or maybe understanding that we might be in active labor soon, promptly fell asleep on the chair. It was nine thirty, and I fell asleep. I had little contractions all night that dilated me to about one or two centimeters. The nurses would check on me and just for fun I'd poke at Eric and tease him in front of the nurses. He continued to sleep and they thought that was all very funny.

By eight the next morning I still hadn't kicked into active labor so they started the Pitocin. Within ten minutes I was in *active labor*. It sure didn't take much.

With Bryna, I had hard contractions but walked through most of my labor. I don't think women realize that there is a trade-off: You get either slow, not terribly painful labor, where you can rest between contractions, or it's *fast*. That's a real gift, but man! Fast means you have to dilate so much quicker. It is a *lot* more painful. It's a much more intense experience than the other kind of labor.

This was Serena's experience. Some women have fast labors that are not a lot more painful than slow ones. But fast labors are usually quite intense, regardless of the pain.

I had already learned from my first pregnancy that birth plans don't work because everything you write down that you don't want in your birth plan is pretty much what you will end up needing. So in my second birth plan, I didn't write things like "I don't want a C-section." But I did write things like "I want to be able to play mellow music, and I want candlelight." When I was in labor, I didn't really care about mellow music, and I sure as hell didn't want candlelight. I wanted my back pushed in a certain way. And I wanted to live through this. The birth plan was silly.

I never considered that this labor would be so intense. But it hit me hard. After I had been on the Pitocin for one hour, Stacey stopped by to see how I was doing. I couldn't believe it was so intense. It was a freight train and it was back labor. They had one of those big inflated medicine balls and I sat on that medicine ball. It was one of the only comforts that I had. My poor husband—he is a really supportive guy and he tries to do as much as he can, but I really didn't want him in my face. That kind of intense labor is the kind where you just suck yourself into your body and all you're doing is concentrating on what's going on from your head down to your toes and then back up to your head and then down through your stomach to your uterus and down to your knees. You're just circling yourself. I mean, *you are in labor* and that's all you can do.

My husband tried to rub me. He tried to pat my hand. He hummed. And all those things were distracting me from being in labor. I thought, "I really appreciate what you're doing, but could you take your lip and put it over your head and get it out of my face?!" And it just got more intense.

I was at three centimeters at about nine thirty and Stacey said, "If you keep going as fast as you're going, you are going to have this baby at about three." And so I was given a focal point! And the clock was right there. A big hospital clock on the wall. I remember looking at that, getting my focal point and saying, "Three. Okay." I think I actually started sectioning off my pain right then and there. I could handle it until three.

But ten o'clock came and I said, "No. No. I cannot handle this pain until three. This pain is too much." So Stacey checked me again and moved it up to one o'clock. I remember thinking, "Okay, one o'clock. I can handle this intense amount of pain until one. I don't know about that. I think maybe not." So I asked if there was someone there to give me an epidural because I thought I couldn't handle that kind of pain for that long.

Once I gave into the fact that I was going to have an epidural, I went into the next stage, and those were the most *intense* contractions. At the time, it was all I could do to be in those contractions. My husband pressed on my lower back and I sat on that ball, and there was nothing I wanted to do but be in that exact position, leaning with my elbows on the bed, my head in my arms and all my weight sitting on the ball. The contractions were about three or four minutes apart. Stacey went out to see about the epidural. Because it was Saturday, there was only one anesthesiologist, and he was in a C-section. They estimated that he would be out by ten thirty and I calculated. "Okay, I can't handle this pain until one, but I can handle it until ten thirty. At ten thirty, relief will come." I was concentrating, living through each contraction. It seemed very odd that I could barely get enough rest through each contraction. But I never thought, "They're coming very, very close now." I had this vision of a slow labor and still didn't even think about a fast one.

People told me lots of stories and I collected them in my head, but I don't think I ever really listened closely to the stories about fast labors. I had already programmed myself that I was having a slow labor. At 10:35 I looked up at the clock and realized that it was five minutes past when he was supposed to be there. I remember saying something to the effect of: "Get that guy! Arrrgh!" Stacey was floating back and forth, checking on me and probably thinking she would just get me the epidural and then come back in a couple of hours. I thought I would have the baby around one thirty even with the epidural. But Stacey, the nurse, and Eric kept coming in at two or three minute intervals, telling me that the anesthesiologist was not done yet, that they were finishing up the C-section and it should be five more minutes.

Five more minutes would pass and I'd say, "*Hello!* Where *is* he?" I asked if Eric could give me the epidural. It didn't seem unreasonable at the time. I was cracking a joke but at the same time I was thinking, "I'm not quite sure why not!" There was a housekeeping person walking by the room. I had seen her on the floor the night before and I knew that she had worked there a long time and she was dressed in scrubs and I figured, "Why not? How hard can an epidural be? It's just giving a shot somewhere. So why have these special people who charge an arm and a leg?" Housekeeping, Eric, my family doc, it didn't matter—anybody could give me an epidural. I didn't care. This whole time I was trying to bargain with Stacey from across the bed. I was still sitting on the medicine ball and still had my elbows on the bed, holding myself up. I thought it was very nice that she came to the other side of the bed and leaned down and looked across at me to talk to me that way.

Once Serena decided to get an epidural, her contractions became less tolerable. This is common. She switched her attention outside her body to the anticipated relief, and this made it more difficult to handle the contractions she continued to have.

I think I was starting to get a little nasty.

I didn't understand why I had to have more pain. It was so much more intense and so much *more*. And then it seemed like the contraction never ended. That was at about ten forty-five. The nurse and Stacey were out of the room. I think neither of them really wanted to talk to me at that point because I was a little crazy.

In the hallway I heard the anesthesiologist and Stacey talking. I heard Stacey's voice distinctively because I was really tuned into my own agenda: "Where's this guy? I need this epidural!" I remember her saying very sweetly to him, "Oh, we've been waiting for you. We have someone who really needs you in here." Very nice. And I remember *him* saying, "Oh. Oh, yeah. I'll take care of that. I've got to run downstairs. I'll be back in about five or ten minutes." And I remember thinking, "*What?* Noooooooooo!"

Anticipating subsequent labors to be like previous ones is a trap. Just as no two children are alike, no two labors are alike. Serena didn't understand why she was in so much discomfort because she didn't know that this labor would be very different from her first and would happen much faster, too.

And that was the point when I turned to Eric and said, "Eric, go get Stacey and ask her if I can go to the toilet because I really, really have to have a bowel movement."

As he was walking out the door, I realized, "This is back labor and it might feel like a bowel movement, but this is the baby." And right when I said that, it clicked. My stomach was doing that same thing, it was already pushing. I didn't have control over it, just like I didn't have control over it with Bryna. I was pushing. And whether I wanted to push or I didn't want to push, that's what was happening. And that's when I said, "Um, Eric, change that. Not bowel movement, baby." And he said, "Oh. *Oh!*" and started running out of the room. I don't know what happened out in the hall but by the time the nurse's head came around the corner, Sophie's head was coming out. And I knew it.

I was just standing next to the bed. I had pushed the ball out of the way. Eric came running in right after the nurse. I decided that I was going to crouch, and he grabbed me under my armpits and pulled me back so that I lost my balance. I think I would have been perfectly happy just standing there having that baby, although Sophie would have had a permanent dent on her head. The nurse started to jump under me while I was still holding onto the bed. When I fell back into Eric's arms, she could get in between me and the bed. Stacey came in. I don't know what happened. It looked like Stacey and the nurse were wrestling for a minute, and I still have a vision of Stacey trying to get under the bed, in her jeans and sneakers, to slide into home. I remember thinking, "This is not baseball!" She caught Sophie just as she came out and I sort of fell back on the floor. Stacey handed her to me immediately.

There Sophie was on my chest and she didn't cry. Her entrance to the world was a lot like her sister's. They didn't really start crying until people started touching them and getting in their faces. They were perfectly fine just to slide out and move on with things. It wasn't until after they had to get pinched, poked, and weighed that they got mad.

I held Sophie for a little bonding moment and then everybody helped me onto the bed because *that's* where you're really supposed to be, *not* the hospital floor! It wasn't the cleanest environment, even if the nurse did throw a towel down first. Stacey cut the cord, and I knew Sophie was fine. She was an old soul from the start, that kid. I know she thought, "Hey, this is kind of fun!" Then we got back up on the bed and the nurse took her to weigh her. I delivered the placenta a few minutes later on the bed. It was very easy. I didn't feel like I needed to do anything else after I had the baby, but Stacey said, "Okay, now you have to push the placenta out." And I thought, "Oh, okay. Whatever. Here. Take that. Let me just deal with this. I have this baby over here and here's your placenta. Whatever." It was a matter of just concentrating and pushing it out. I didn't really care about that. I cared about the baby. They handed Sophie to me and I nursed her for awhile.

That anesthesiologist pushed me over the edge. He made me really mad. He came in right about ten minutes after Sophie was born. Stacey turned to him and said, "We don't need you. Thank you anyway." And I said, "Yeah, yeah. Thanks for nothing." I thought it was wickedly humorous that he could just say, "I'm going to take a little break before I take care of that."

Sophie was a very mellow baby from the start. She weighed seven pounds, three ounces. The funny thing about it is I'm pretty sure she's been smiling since the day she was born. I just don't buy that it's a reflex—not when your three-hour-old baby looks up at you and smiles.

I didn't need stitches. I just had a little stinging. After Bryna, I couldn't believe how bruised I felt down there; it hurt when I peed. But with Sophie, my body

After hours in surgery, the anesthesiologist needed to take care of some personal needs before he jumped right into another delicate procedure. This was understandable, but Serena was focused on that epidural being her salvation. She was so distracted by the promised epidural that she didn't notice that she was ready to deliver her baby.

recovered so much quicker. Once those cells were reawakened, they said, "Oh yeah, yeah, yeah. Birth. Remember that? We did that a couple of years ago."

The Pitocin worked like it was supposed to. It kicked me into labor, which is a whole different concept than needing it to keep your labor going. It was pretty intense. Even though I've never had a natural contraction, I could tell there were two different types: the completely synthetic ones, where the Pitocin was forcing the contraction completely. Those were a lot easier to take. But the contractions that the Pitocin kicked in, the ones that combined with my own hormones, were so much more quick and intense. I went pretty much from one to ten in a matter of three hours, which was a wee bit painful.

Whatever you do, whatever happens, going through labor is worth it. And it's just one day. It's only one day in your life. And if you trust your doctor, your spouse, and yourself, it will be fine. You can't prepare for the unwanted things because then they become the things you focus on. You just have to prepare to be surprised. And know your stuff. Know what "placenta previa" is and all of those things. Know what they are, but don't obsess about them.

One of the biggest lessons I learned from birth and from children is that I don't have control. And if you're a person that needs control over every aspect, it's not going to be pleasant for you. It will be a struggle the whole time. But if you're willing to accept that sometimes you don't have control, it can be a very pleasant experience. That's the same with raising children. You can control whether or not your children have manners, but you can't control their personalities. You can't control their likes and dislikes. That is true with birth. It is only one day and you're going to have to give up some control. I'm not saying give up control to the doctor. I'm not saying give up control to a bossy or even a particularly sweet nurse. And I'm not saying give up control to your husband. I'm saying give up control over your expectations.

This is why the birth plan was a total joke. It really doesn't matter about the birth. It matters about the baby. That one day is amazing and what it does is humbling and humiliating and exhilarating and strengthening. What really comes out of it is your baby, which is what really matters. And the birth part of it? Who cares how it happens?

There's not that much that you can say when you have this little baby running around the park and you stand next to this other mom and you both invariably start talking about birth and she says, "Oh, I couldn't do it. I had an epidural." And she has this beautiful child. And you say, "Well, I did it all natural." Both of you have a miracle running around, playing in the park. And they are both amazing.

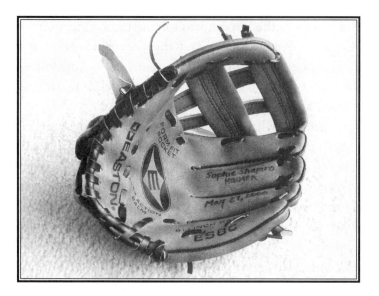

TEN POUNDS, FOURTEEN OUNCES

LARA AND JOSEPH

There is nothing like a strong, respectful, and supportive relationship to ease the birth process. Lara's husband, Serge, provided loving support throughout her pregnancy and labor. Add a strong dose of faith, and you have an excellent recipe for a good birth.

I am not in the least bit particular about the brand of faith my patients embrace. I can accommodate any religion, any set of beliefs, and any positive support system a woman brings to a birth. If the family is Christian, I welcome Jesus and Mother Mary. If they are pagan, I welcome the Goddess. I am thrilled to have Spirit consciously represented in any of Her forms.

Lara and Serge are Greek Orthodox. I had no idea prior to this birth that they were so active in their church; it had never come up during our prenatal visits. When I walked into the room at the hospital to induce Lara, I saw her icons on the window sill. I asked about them and she explained the strength she gained from their presence. I breathed a sigh of relief, knowing we would be attended by Spirit for the next several hours.

Lara and Serge's first baby, Joseph Seraphim, weighed ten pounds, fourteen ounces. He was probably the largest baby I ever delivered vaginally in a hospital. We induced Lara's labor when she was over two weeks late. Lara's belly was huge, and the baby was obviously ready. Lara was in complete agreement with our plan to induce.

Fortunately, all I had to do was break her membranes to get things started. I had anticipated needing to use Prostin gel next to her cervix and then perhaps IV Pitocin later, but Lara was having little contractions when she showed up at the hospital. We simply helped her labor along.

Because this baby was so large and was Lara's first, and the birth canal was traumatized more than usual by his passage, we had to do some extensive stitching after the birth. But Lara was remarkably calm and positive throughout the procedure, and even sang to her husband as I and another doctor stitched away.

Assisting and watching Lara give birth was an honor. Her love for her husband and this new baby, her faith, her courage, and her priorities were all crystal clear. She never lost sight of her priorities, and her spiritual integrity was better than any drug I could have offered her.

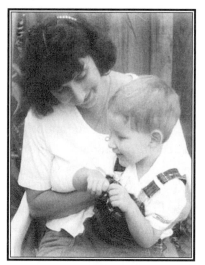

Lara and Joseph

LARA: Joseph was born on June 8th, 1996. I started the Bradley classes in April—late like everything else. My few anxious moments were eased by those classes. Serge was very supportive during the pregnancy. I worked for about seven months, and Serge would make dinner, clean the house, and do laundry, and he would always tell me I was beautiful and how wonderful I looked. He really tried to understand what I was going through.

About two weeks before the due date, I was really anxious and excited. I didn't know what the contractions would be like, or how I would know. I thought that I was going to have back labor because my back ached in the evenings. But because he was almost three weeks late, after a week or two I thought, "I don't care. *Any way* he comes; it's just fine." I stopped answering my phone because people would say, "Is he here yet? Is he here yet?"

My Mom was here for five weeks! She came a week before his due date to help me. We sat here in the morning, and I drank milk and then put the cup on my stomach because he would kick. That's how we would entertain ourselves. We were so bored. Everything was done. All the bills were paid and in order. All the groceries were bought.

And then because he was so late, it all fell apart again. I had packed my bags to be prepared for a long, lengthy labor. When I was packing, Serge said, "What are you bringing all these books for?" I replied, "In case you get bored. I don't know. How do I know it's not going to end up being a Caesarian and then I'm in the hospital for a week? I want books." So I packed everything, including oatmeal cookies.

We finally had to break the water to induce me, and in a way I was glad the baby was going to be here, but I really wanted that experience of waking up in the middle of the night: "Oh I think this is it!"

Serge thinks Joseph was late because he takes after me. I'm late with everything! But I think it was because I was eating so well. I was on 100 grams of protein a day. When he was a week overdue I said, "Forget this. I just can't eat this much any more." Everything I ate was protein-rich food. I think he just had it too good in there. He was just too happy, cozy, and well fed.

He was due on Tuesday, May 21ˢᵗ. Two weeks later, my doctor said, "Well, let's get an ultrasound to make sure he's all right." He was perfectly fine. The technician who did the test said, "Oh, he'll be about eight and a half pounds." I thought, "Oh, okay. That's fine. No problem." That was Wednesday. Friday I came in for a checkup and she said, "All right, this is long enough." I agreed. So we made an appointment for three thirty that afternoon at the hospital so that I could be monitored and they could put some gel inside—which, as it turned out, we didn't have to do.

Lara had the opportunity to refuse induction. Her baby was still doing well, but no one wanted to wait until he was showing signs of distress. When I brought up the possibility of inducing her, she listened to all the pros and cons and decided she wanted to make it happen. She was in control of this decision.

I was late for the appointment because the neighbor's house in the back was getting broken into. Serge called 911 thinking it would be quick, but she kept him on the line and he said, "Look, I have to go. My wife has to go to the hospital to have her baby." So she thought I was in labor. The whole time she was asking, "Is she all right? Is she all right?" And I was just thinking, "Come on, come on." But anyway, that diverted our minds. My mother was so anxious. We were really laughing about the whole thing on the way to the hospital. I was really in a happy mood, just laughing and thinking, "Yeah, this is just perfect, being late as usual."

When the nurses hooked me up they said, "You're having contractions." And I said, "I am? I don't feel anything." I was really excited. I know the nurse checked my cervix, but I don't remember if she said I was dilated or what. At that point, my belly was so big, Serge wanted to write on it and say, "Help! Let me out!" He begged me and begged me and said he would cook dinner for a year if I'd let him. He wrote it right under my belly button, near where the fetal monitor goes because he wanted the nurse to see it. He cooked dinner for the first six weeks of Joe's life, and that was good enough.

So I had started contractions, and they were regular enough, but they weren't strong enough. Around six o'clock my doctor came in and broke my membranes, which were really tough—all that protein. It made Serge nervous, but I kept saying, "I don't feel anything. Don't worry!"

I got up and we went for a walk. It was very uncomfortable. I was thinking as I got up, "Okay, how do I adjust to this situation? I'm going to be leaking everywhere. I am not going to walk down the hall leaking everywhere and slipping and whatever." But the nurse gave me a pad and we walked. We went to see the babies already in the nursery. Some friends came to visit, found us in the hallway, and I started to have contractions that I could feel.

I was excited and I'd say, "Okay, here comes one," and everyone would watch. It wasn't that bad; it was just cramps. I was trying to drink so I wouldn't get dehydrated because I didn't want an IV in me. We went out on the patio to walk, and Serge set up a little route for me. He put chairs in an obstacle course and said, "Okay, you've got to walk around the chairs and the cone."

I was getting contractions about every five minutes at this point. I could get around the course twice, and then they'd start up again. It was starting to get more intense. They weren't really hurting, but they were definitely there. And so I'd lean on Serge and just breathe and relax. I remember this specifically: I walked around twice, and that happened. Then I walked around once and it happened again. I walked around again and could barely make it around. They happened again, and I said, "I want to go back to the room now. *Now*." And I never left the room after that until Joseph was born.

I went into the shower. I don't remember a whole lot, but Serge says I was revitalized after the shower. I love showers anyway. I love water, so it felt really nice. There was a chair right there in the shower, and the funny thing was that Serge accidentally pulled the emergency cord. And within seconds, the nurse was there. And I thought, "Good. They're very responsive." My room was right next to the nurse's station.

Then I went to bed, and the contractions got stronger. I don't remember how dilated my cervix was then. In all the books, they said that sometimes if you are slow to dilate, it can be frustrating. So I don't think I even wanted to know. I wasn't paying much attention to that, but I think at this point we were creating ambiance in the room. We put music on: Mozart, Prague Symphonies, and Beethoven. Joe was born to Mozart. We put up icons—the icon of the Mother of God, and Saint Ann, who was Mary's mother—because I knew they'd been through it, and they could help me. Any time it got very difficult, when it really got intense and I felt like I didn't have control, that's when I would pray. I would look at the icons and say, "Help me. Help me." And repeating that really worked. In fact, before the intensity started, Serge and I said the "Our Father" together.

Lara was reassured by the nursing staff. She wanted to be in the hospital with nurses to help when needed.

I expected it to hurt more, but it was just bad cramps. It was not unrecognizable pain. I have a high tolerance for pain; I have a high tolerance for a lot of things. I can adjust to things. Maybe I'm just lazy, and I don't want to do anything about it. But it seems to help. When I was in high school, I used to have bad periods and stay home for two or three days. So that feeling was not unfamiliar to me and with that kind of pain,

I know how to relax and just let go. So I was surprised. I wasn't going to say anything to anybody about it because I thought, "The minute I say something, it's going to get really bad." But through the whole labor it felt like bad cramps. That could be painful to some people, but it wasn't for me.

I didn't want any medicine. I knew I wasn't going to be unreason-able about it, but it would have to be some severe sharp pain for a long period of time before I would take medicine. Or, maybe I would have taken medicine if the pain was sapping my strength. But no, I didn't require it. I don't even take aspirin for a headache or cramps. I would just go and lie down.

Transition was a fun one. I think when I hit transition, the baby had dropped and I was inclined on my back. The nurses came up to me and had me roll over. I knew something was wrong because all of the sudden they put the oxygen mask on me and wanted to insert the internal fetal monitor. So I thought to myself, "Something must be wrong, but I can't panic. That's their job. They can do whatever they need to do. I need to relax. Because that's what I can do about this situation."

Sometimes when the baby enters the birth canal, the heart rate will show a brief period of stress. Changing the mother's position and supplying extra oxygen can help the baby recover quickly. The internal fetal monitor was interventional, but Lara did not mind. She focused on the work of giving birth and perceived the medical interventions as helpful rather than invasive.

They turned me over on my hands and knees so that I was leaning over the back of the bed, and then they inserted the fetal monitor. I guess when he dropped, his heart rate went down, but he recovered really quickly. And I actually liked the oxygen mask because I have a little bit of asthma and sometimes have a hard time breathing. At that point, I assumed that this was the transition, because from then on I was pushing.

What happened with the contractions was that I threw up every time. The first time it really startled me because I wasn't expecting it. I mean, I threw up *every* single time, every three to five minutes for two or three hours. I remember my doctor warming up the baby bed, and that gave me energy and excitement again. And the whole time I was looking at the clock. I swore I wouldn't do that, but I kept doing it because everything seemed to be going so quickly. And I said, "Wow! Wow! This is great!" But the throwing up. . . My first thought was that I had just made a wonderful lunch before we went to the hospital. I had been craving red peppers the whole time I was pregnant, and when I threw up, I thought, "They're going to think it's blood." I remember saying to Serge in a feeling of panic, "You know that craving for red peppers I had? I don't think I'm going to have it anymore." That made everyone laugh. So when I tell people how my labor was, I say it was like a bad flu: cramping and throwing up. Serge would bring the little basin and say, "Here's your little friend," and I wanted to slug him.

It took a while to learn how to push. Vomiting was so surprising and uncomfortable that it was difficult to concentrate on pushing. At one point, I think I'd been pushing for about an hour, and my doctor told me, "Okay, just breathe and relax and don't push for a few contractions." "Okay, fine, great, great." And by not pushing for a few times, I realized the urge to push—by not doing it. So then it was easier to work with it. But boy, I was in every position: with the squatting bar, with my leg up, with just about everything.

Women will sometimes vomit during labor. The midwives tell us that as a woman opens up at one end by vomiting, she will also open up at the other, so vomiting can actually be helpful. It may be uncomfortable, but not dangerous.

I had been pushing for about three hours when my doctor said she wanted to use the vacuum suction cup. I remember coming to, and saying, "Will that hurt the baby?" And she said, "Not if I don't use it for very long." So she waited for a couple of more pushes and I really, for the life of me, tried. And I just couldn't. I just couldn't.

She hooked up the vacuum suction cup, and it was uncomfortable. I'd say the only pain I felt was that burning sensation—that's the best way to describe it. It felt like someone set me on fire, like the Johnny Cash song, "Ring of Fire." That's what it was. I knew I was almost there and that it wasn't going to be another hour. Again, knowing what goes on in the process of birth really helps. Because even if you're out of it for most of it, when you recognize these signs, they're really encouraging.

I didn't want an episiotomy. All the women I'd ever talked to who had had episiotomies said they still felt them. And my sister-in-law, who's had five children, said that with the first one she had an episiotomy, and then with the second one, she tore where the episiotomy was. And that she still feels it. But we just didn't know how big he was going to be!

DR. KERR: Lara did not get an episiotomy, but she did need the help of the vacuum suction cup on Joseph's head to accomplish her delivery. The little cup attached with suction to the baby's head and when she pushed, I pulled to help move the baby out. There are risks associated with using this device, but done correctly and for no more than three contractions, the benefits outweigh the risks. After three push-pulls, together we eased him out.

Although episiotomies used to be a routine part of medically managed deliveries, it is now understood that they are usually not helpful. On the other hand, while it may make the first few days of recovery more difficult, most women do heal completely and have no long term negative effects from an episiotomy.

LARA: I remember him coming completely out. I was thinking the whole time that first his head would come out and I'd have to give a couple more pushes, and he just— boom. There. I saw him on me and I said, "Oh, thank goodness. This is over." But at the same time I was thinking of women who'd say to me, "Oh, I'd do it all over again." And I immediately thought, "It wasn't that bad." That's what I said.

It felt comfortable having him there. At the same time, I really wanted to rest.

I didn't know if he was a boy or a girl. I hadn't even thought to look. I just thought, "Oh good, the baby's here." Someone told me he was a boy; I didn't look. But as soon as he was born, I quit throwing up.

I knew they had to push on your belly afterwards, but Oh God did she push. That was getting the clots out. The placenta was easy, only one or two pushes. It felt good. It was very *warm*.

I didn't even think about his size. I was just happy he was there. He didn't cry. It was amazing. Just how on earth did that miracle happen? Wow! It was 1:17 on Saturday morning, and he surprised us all by weighing ten pounds, fourteen ounces!

I needed a few stitches—not many—and that didn't hurt. It went really smoothly. They put an IV in, but I didn't care. The nurse was very, very nice. She kept coming in and checking my stitches. I was exhausted but still excited, so I wasn't sleeping at that point. I was asking all kinds of questions about Joe. He was in the nursery, and they were cleaning him and doing his footprints and that sort of thing.

At this particular hospital, most laboring women got IVs. A woman can negotiate the need for that protocol if she does not want it and if there is no clear reason for the IV line.

Then the nurse noticed a lump near my stitches. She kept pressing on it and it kept getting bigger and bigger. I didn't feel it, but when she touched it I could feel something. She said, "This doesn't look good, so I'm just going to call the doctor." And again I knew that whatever it was, that if I remained calm, that would be the best situation. Because, again, that was *my* job. I couldn't do anything else to help.

This hospital had a nursery separate from the mothers' rooms. Some women appreciate having the nurses watch their babies while they get some rest after the delivery. If you want your baby with you at all times, you need to make sure the hospital policy will accommodate your wishes.

DR. KERR: Lara had developed some bleeding under the surface of her vagina. This can happen when a very large baby comes through the birth canal. We needed to take out the original stitches, find the source of the bleeding, and pack it with sterile gauze. This was a two-person job because of the location, and at that point I called in another doctor to help me do the repair.

LARA: Serge was worried. My doctor had to call in another doctor. Serge got scrubs on, and they moved me to the operating room. There was a blood clot, and they had to unstitch and then restitch me. I thought, "Okay. Whatever." But Serge is very protective and he wants everything just so and gets worried if it isn't. I know that.

In fact, all through the labor, Serge didn't know what was going on because he was not in my position, and I couldn't always communicate. I couldn't sit there and have a conversation, so I'd wink, and that way he knew everything was all right. He said he really liked that: "Wink means I'm okay. I may look intense, but I'm okay."

Going to the operating room I was half concerned about Joe. But again I really relied on the staff, and I felt comfortable with them. I was given some sort of medicine (Nubain), but I was awake, which I liked. I didn't want to be knocked out. I remember the whole procedure as very uncomfortable. The pain was like when you have a cat on your lap with claws and it starts to knead. But it wasn't my legs it was kneading. It was that kind of small, sharp and quick pain but not unbearable. But I was saying, "Oooooowww. Ooooooowwww. Oooooowww." Serge didn't like that, but making those sounds helped me. Then I realized he was not doing well.

I had the icon next to my face there in the operating room with Serge on the other side. I wanted to calm him, so I started singing and humming, and he said, "What song is that?" I didn't know the words until I got to the chorus, so I said, "You'll hear in a minute." And I kept humming so he really had to concentrate. Hold on, just listen to the song. And then I sang, "Funiculi, funiculae," so that he could sing along. I think that kind of lightened the mood. It let him know, "Look, I'm all right. This is just what we gotta do right now." I didn't even want to think about the stitches. I just didn't want to think about it. The packing going in there was uncomfortable. I didn't want it to get lost in me.

DR. KERR: As the other doctor and I worked on Lara's vagina, the

Complications can be much easier to handle if you're able to accept the unexpected and if you're not trying to do it alone. This couple really knew how to take care of each other.

scene was surreal. We were at one end dealing with sutures, blood, and packing, and Lara was singing to her husband on the other side of the drapes. At that moment the operating room was a very sweet space. Her faith and love permeated that high-tech medical world.

LARA: I remember getting a little shaky. I didn't feel sick. I felt tired. And I remember watching the clock on the wall. It was about an hour for the whole procedure.

After that, the only pain that was really uncomfortable was in my back, because of the throwing up. It was like recovering from a really bad flu. My stomach ached from throwing up, and my back was sore.

I remember everyone being very impressed by how much Joe weighed. But it was a novelty that wore off very quickly because during every new nurse's shift, they'd come in to introduce themselves and say, "You're the one, you poor thing. How are you doing?" And they were good, but they were too much. I thought, "Humph. It's done. I'm fine. Don't say it to me that way. I'm okay." I just wanted to make sure that the stitching and everything was doing all right.

That night Serge stayed on a little bed they brought in for him. When the nurse came in at midnight to wake me up to take all my vitals, I knew: "I'm not getting any rest here. I want to go home." The next day they took out the packing and I went home.

Home with Joe—the first week after my mother left—nothing got done. When Serge came home he'd say, "How are you doing?" And I'd say, "I brushed my teeth today!" And that was it. I just did what the baby wanted. He came home one time and found me crying. I was holding Joseph and he said, "What's wrong?" I remember saying, "I don't want him to go away to college. I want him to stay with me." He said, "We've got plenty of time to worry about that." But I remember Joseph was so beautiful, so wonderful, that I didn't want him ever to leave me. I knew in my head that this was ridiculous, but. . .

If I could give advice to someone else, I would say that if you are taking a birthing class, get the facts but don't get caught up in all the hype. Understand the physical processes that happen. Don't get disappointed if it doesn't go the way you wanted it to. Be prepared for whatever, and go with the flow. That's just it. Know what to expect, physically, and just go with it.

After this birth I started paying closer attention to what my pregnant patients were eating. Plenty of protein is good, but too much is too much of a good thing! Lara's next baby was smaller than Joseph and came quickly. I was at a Halloween party when Lara called to say she was in labor. I sent her to the hospital to be checked, but I stayed at the party, remembering how long it had taken her to birth Joseph. An hour later I got a call to come quickly, and five minutes after I ran in, dressed as a tie-dye hippie from the '70s, Moses was born. Lara had no complications with this second son's birth or with her daughter, who arrived two years later. She is truly one of the best baby-havers I know!

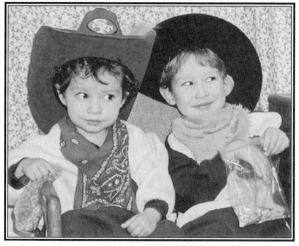

Moses and Joseph

HAVING HOLDEN

HEATHER AND HOLDEN

Heather is a very sensitive and smart woman. A lawyer by trade, she is also an alcoholic with over fifteen years of sobriety. She considers her sobriety birthday her true birthday. She is the first to tell you that staying sober is not easy. She is logical and linear, intelligent and introverted, with strong emotions that run deep. Her experience with people and her self-knowledge allow her to tell her own birth story with unusual clarity and insight.

Heather had wonderfully normal births. But postpartum depression hit hard after each one. After her first baby, it took her months to figure out what was wrong. This was supposed to be the most wonderful time of her life and she was overwhelmingly sad. Then she felt guilty because she was sad. She was afraid to tell anyone how she felt; it was too inappropriate. When Alex was well over a year old, she finally realized that she was significantly depressed in spite of her "perfect family."

Heather was the first patient I ever gave a written prescription for a personal retreat. She went to the northern Pacific coast for three days and allowed herself to grieve the loss of her previous self. She would never be the same. She was now a mother, and her life required her to give up much of her own self to her child and her marriage. By honoring that transition, she came to a place of peace and understanding. She returned from that retreat with a certainty that she did not want any more children. Her one perfect Alex was enough.

Eventually, Heather and Ted did decide to have another child, and Heather found herself falling in love all over again. Her life will never be simple, but she handles it with grace and integrity. I find her an inspiration to all women who wonder why they ever decided to give up their independence and have demanding and delightful babies. We become so vulnerable when we become mothers. Heather knows this well.

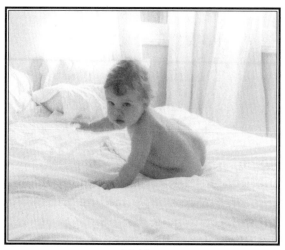

Holden

HEATHER: This was my second pregnancy—one I was not sure about, nor completely comfortable with. With my first pregnancy, I was so excited and in awe of what was happening to my body that I pretty much ignored what was happening in my life. We moved. Ted changed jobs. I quit my career to be the perfect mom. We lived about two thousand miles from the nearest relative and knew no one.

We had a textbook natural birth at a freestanding birth center. When I was seven months pregnant, we had switched to midwives from an arrogant obstetrician who scheduled Cesarean sections whenever he was going on vacation so that he could "be there" for the mother. At the birth center, we had great support in a nurturing environment, and I was sure that our perfect birth was a sign that everything was going to work out just as I had imagined.

After Alex was born, I discovered how exhausting, boring, and mind numbing caring for a small baby was. I was absolutely in love with him. But I had no help and no friends and was completely overwhelmed most of the time. I resented the fact that my husband just got up, showered, grabbed his keys and left for his day, his life virtually untouched by our new son. My life consisted of sitting and holding and nursing the baby, who was virtually unputdownable. I slipped quietly, and not so quietly, into depression. I felt horrid for not loving every minute, and I could not understand what had happened at what was supposed to be one of the most wonderful times of my life.

About a year and a half after seeking counseling and having rashes, assorted unspecified illnesses, panic attacks, short-term memory loss, and hot and cold flashes—and ultimately feeling like a complete failure as a mother and a person—my doctor and I finally figured out that I had postpartum depression. I started with antidepressants and a three-day vacation to Sea Ranch in northern California, which gave me solitude and allowed me to sleep. (It was prescribed by my doctor).

When I finally felt a little better, I confessed to my husband that I was not going to have any more children. Ted's reaction was my worst nightmare. He insisted that I had promised to have two children. If I couldn't perform on my promise, he was not sure he wanted to stay married to me. More counseling. I had been asking myself whether I thought I could manage, or at least survive, having another baby. That answer was almost always no, and therefore I was not having another baby.

After six more months, I was able to see past my fear and ask myself again if I wanted to have another baby. I decided I would like Alex to have a sibling, I was pretty sure I would like to stay married to Ted, and if I could avoid the depression, I would like another child.

Everyone assured me it would be different this time. I could stay on antidepressants through the pregnancy. We now had friends, neighbors, babysitters and a great preschool. And I had an incredible part-time job working with wonderful people who saw me as an intelligent, talented person. I would not get depressed. Everything was going to be okay.

So I got pregnant again.

Heather was taking an antidepressant that had shown no adverse side effects on babies or children. We discussed her options and together agreed that her mental state was very important for both her and her baby. She chose to continue her medication so she would not be dangerously depressed during her pregnancy.

That pregnancy flew by. I was busy with work and Alex, who was by then almost three years old. I had done it once, so everything was less amazing and noteworthy. I had survived the first one, so my husband figured I did not really need any special attention. He rarely attended the doctors' appointments. Instead, Alex, Dr. Kerr, and I had a great time listening to the baby, listening to Alex, measuring my tummy with the frog measuring tape, and measuring and weighing Alex. The best part was how excited Alex was about having a new baby and how cool he thought my expanding tummy was.

When I was around seven or eight months pregnant, Dr. Kerr had to remind me that growing a new life was an important, full-time job, and that perhaps it was time to pay attention to getting some rest and taking care of myself. She told me I was in denial about being pregnant. I was.

I was also in no hurry to have the baby. I knew it was easier to take care of a baby while it was still inside. But eventually, I became big enough and uncomfortable enough to look forward to holding the little guy who kept kicking me.

I went into labor on a Monday. I started having some contractions, knew what they were, and wasn't really concerned. That afternoon, things started to pick up a bit. Ted and I walked around the block and to the grocery store. By that evening the contractions were getting closer together. But I was tired and didn't really want to be up all night in labor. So I took a nice warm bath and everything stopped. I went to bed at eight thirty and slept all night.

The next morning, I got up, ate breakfast, and we started walking again. Within an hour of starting to walk, the contractions picked up where they left off. We called the doctor to let her know it was the real thing. We ran some

Heather was in early latent labor. Real active labor will not stop with warm baths or sleep. That's one way to know if it's active labor: Try to stop the contractions when you need to get some rest. And it's important to get rest during latent labor. Allow your body to quietly do all the early work while you continue to store up energy for the big push to come.

errands and kept walking. At this point, the contractions were strong enough that I did not want to walk too far from home. Besides, I had to go to the bathroom every fifteen minutes, so I could not go too far anyway.

So we just walked around the block. It was the most wonderful time. All our friends and neighbors came out to talk to us, to wish the baby safe passage, and to bless my belly. I felt so connected to life and to the love of other people for me and the baby.

The day progressed. So did the contractions. We had friends pick up Alex at his school and keep him overnight. I ate something for dinner. I think it was pizza. Ted and I thumbed through baby-name books. (We knew it was a boy, but Ted did not see any point in naming the baby until he was actually here.) I was starting to turn inward. I only half-heard conversations. I could talk but didn't really feel like it. During the early evening, the contractions became more intense. We called Dr. Kerr to check in. Then it was eight o'clock and everything stopped again. It was baby's bedtime and my bedtime. So I slept again.

When I woke up and started moving around again, the contractions came back. Our next-door neighbor rode his skateboard to the bakery for chocolate croissants and brought me a large decaf cappuccino. (We had delivered pizza to them two weeks earlier when they were in labor.) Then we walked some more. Our friends smiled and waved and wished us well, laughing because we were still walking around the block in labor. Ted and I finally agreed on a name: Holden. It means deep valley in old English, and we both just liked it.

At some point late in the morning, my water broke. I remember going through at least two pairs of pants, thinking I had very poor bladder control. Then I recognized the smell of the amniotic fluid and realized I couldn't shut it off. I hate wearing sanitary pads. But at that point, I did not really care.

Around noon on Wednesday, things started to rock and roll. There are "walking around" contractions and then there are "I don't care if I'm in the middle of an intersection during rush hour, I'm not moving" contractions. I was starting to get the second kind. I remember spending a lot of time holding on to the mantle of the fireplace, which seemed to be just the right height.

What a difference attitude and perception makes! Knowing that each contraction is helping, and knowing that each one will end, makes the whole process bearable.

I also remember feeling a lot more calm and assured than with my first labor. This time I understood that every contraction really would end. During my first labor, I wasn't ever sure. I was scared of the pain and resistant to the contractions because I was uncomfortable and did not know how long I could last. This time I knew that every contraction was helping get it over with; and I knew I could last.

I still had to go to the bathroom a lot. My bladder would relax and I would have another contraction. Ted sat on the bathtub while I sat on the toilet and held his knees. I was very focused and had little sense of time or what was going on around me. I remember thinking it must have been a while because Ted kept saying, "You're doing great" over and over and over. At about four thirty in the afternoon, I was ready to go to the hospital. I wanted to be done with labor. Ted called the doctor and told her I needed to be around someone with a new voice and a new face.

I did not go back to the birth center because the birth center had revoked all the MDs' privileges. It was more important for me to have my doctor at the birth than to be at the birth center. She was my doctor—my children's doctor—and she had saved my life when I was struggling with postpartum depression after Alex was born. I needed her because she was the one I trusted to help me when I was most vulnerable.

So we drove to the hospital. Luckily it was only a few blocks away, because having contractions while strapped into a seatbelt sucks. We made sure to pack Holden's present to Alex, a new scooter, so that Holden could give it to him.

I had several "don't care if I'm in the middle of the street" contractions walking into the hospital. I remember seeing photographs of men in suits lining the hallway. They were all smiling at me. I found this extremely annoying. We had preregistered and so went straight to the labor and delivery department.

We were met by a nurse named Shannon. She had already talked to Dr. Kerr, was expecting us, and knew that we had done a lot of work at home.

*Heather refused contin-
uous monitoring and
had absolutely no
interventions during her
birth. She had no IV, no
internal monitors, and no
medications. That's the
way she wanted it, and
there was no reason to do
it any differently.*

She took us straight into the delivery room. She asked me to put on a really big ace bandage over my belly. This was the fetal monitor. I didn't really want a fetal monitor but agreed to at least put it on. After the first contraction with the monitor, I was done being tied to machines, especially ones with strings to keep straight.

I was most comfortable on my hands and knees, holding onto the raised head of the bed. The change of environment and my fear of hospitals increased my discomfort level, so I asked Shannon to call Dr. Kerr and tell her I needed her. Shannon came back to tell me she had called and asked Dr. Kerr to come, and she was already on her way. Right then, as if by magic, Dr. Kerr walked in the door. I felt better and knew I was going to be okay.

I labored awhile sitting on an exercise ball and holding onto the bed with Ted supporting me from the back. The change of position was good. Then I just felt cranky and ready to get it over with. I told Dr. Kerr that I had about had it and that I just wanted to get this baby out of me. She said it sounded a bit like transition and checked to see if I was fully

*Having your birth
team around you,
calmly supporting you
and being optimistic,
can help you overcome
the stress of changing
environments and
your fear of the
hospital.*

dilated. I had some scar tissue on my cervix from treatment for dysplasia years ago. It refused to stretch out with my first baby and was refusing again. Dr. Kerr held the stubborn bit through several contractions to tuck it behind the baby's head. After that I could push and really felt the baby start to move.

At some point during my first labor, I had learned to push. This time, my body remembered, although I still tried to pull away from some of the contractions. I got up to squat on the edge of the bed to shorten the distance to "out." Shannon attached a bar over the bed to hold onto. This really helped. With every push, there was a lot of excitement. Ted and Dr. Kerr and Shannon would yell, "Come on, come on, keep going!" I just felt relief that we were coming to the end. It seemed like I had a million contractions while everyone was saying that they could see the baby's head. Ted took my hand and helped me touch Holden's squishy wet hair. Another contraction. More yelling. "Keep going!" "The head is out." "Keep going. Keep going. Keep going. You're almost there." Then came the shoulder, and then relief. Holden was on my chest and Shannon was rubbing him with a warm blanket and clearing his nose with the little blue suction ball. The first thing I noticed was his round little bottom and chubby legs. He looked at me and looked around and then found my nipple. Ted cut the cord. Holden was born at 7:20 p.m.

After a while, Dr. Kerr weighed and measured Holden. Nine pounds, twelve ounces. He was much bigger than any of us expected. Now we understood why my body needed a couple of days to warm up for this delivery. Holden kept making little "uh, uh uh" sounds and looked around. We called and asked our friends to bring Alex to the hospital. Alex was so excited. He helped clean Holden's poop off my belly and helped me eat some dinner. Then Ted and Alex went home and Holden and I went to bed. By this time it was after ten and way past our bedtime.

Heather's world is very full with two sons that are the light of her life and a career as partner in a law firm. She continues to juggle her career demands, the demands of a family, and her own personal needs.

Heather told me that she believes our society would benefit if we honored the mother of a newborn and allowed her to grieve the loss of her former self when we celebrate her becoming a new mother. Not every new mother is upset by these transitions, but most feel the loss of freedom and have conflicting feelings about that loss. They feel guilty for their "selfish" thoughts and try to deny their own needs so they can be the best mothers they can be. Heather teaches us that loving your child unconditionally is important, but loving yourself enough to honor your own true feelings makes you the best mother you could possibly be.

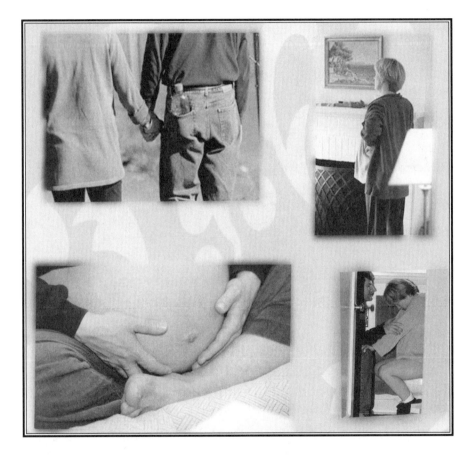

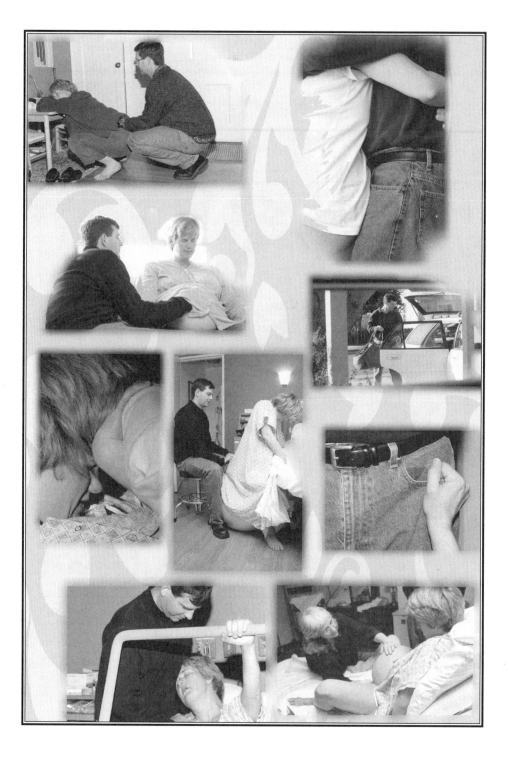

POSTGRADUATE TRAINING

RENEE AND OLIVER

Renee, a family physician, and Veronica, a practicing osteopath, are a loving and committed couple who decided to have a baby together. Though Renee had delivered many babies for her patients, this was her first pregnancy. She saw it as an extension of her ongoing education in medicine.

Renee's birthing process blends her natural tendency for intellectual observation with a pure, unthinking birth experience. When Oliver was born, five doctors shared the joy: Renee and her partner, two supportive friends including myself, and the physician delivering the baby. We created a party, and we were perfectly comfortable celebrating Oliver's birth in the hospital.

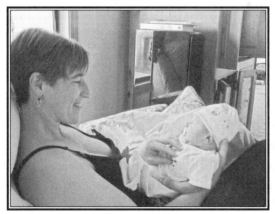

Renee and Oliver

RENEE: I didn't have to think too long and hard about choosing a provider for my pregnancy. As a health care provider myself, I knew most of the delivering physicians and midwives in the community, and

I wanted to have someone I knew I could just be myself with. I wanted someone I knew enough about that I could be completely trusting.

I had an experience in my training with an obstetrician who trusted me at an early stage in my education. That was a very important moment, and she got my respect right away. It turns out that this physician was also very sensitive to my particular situation of being with a woman. She is also an openly lesbian woman who has gone through the process of getting pregnant and delivering. She's into most forms of birth, she works with midwives, and I thought she would be willing to work with me, whatever I wanted. She has an open mind and she can communicate.

I didn't think seriously about going to a birth center with midwives because of my age. I was forty when I got pregnant. I realized I was at greater risk of potential complications. Having never given birth before, I might have a prolonged or difficult labor. And the thought of being in my home made me a little bit anxious—probably because I work in health care and I've seen all the things that can happen. To me, being in the health care setting was not a foreign environment. It wasn't as if the hospital was a strange place. I almost felt as if it was home, because I'd spent so many hours of my life there. I would be safe in the hospital, and I could just be myself and be open to whatever I could learn.

I had to let go of fear. I didn't want to hold on to the worry that if something was wrong, there wouldn't be a place to tend to it or someone who could tend to it. Not that I felt a lot of fear. I have to say I wasn't fearful that something would go wrong; I just didn't want that to be part of the picture.

I thought of my pregnancy as a unique educational opportunity for me to really understand pregnancy, labor, and delivery—better than I could ever understand it even being right there with women, during intense moments, as a delivering family physician. I thought, "I want to work with someone who could potentially give me further instructions beyond what I would otherwise get."

I did have the expectation that my nursing staff would be respectful and understanding of my requests, the same as when I'm the working physician. I had the expectation that my physician would work with me and be open, and I had the expectation that my labor and delivery was going to be very hard. I've seen many women in that position, struggling with what turned out to be the most difficult thing they'd ever done.

I had had a very early ultrasound that wasn't official, just to show there was just one baby. My partner is a doctor and she did it. We had our first formal ultrasound at nineteen weeks, which looked good.

We had an abnormal blood test—the result of a special test that was done because of my age. It was a combination of blood work and an ultrasound. There was one abnormal result in the blood that could've possibly been a problem, but I decided, based on the ultrasound, that the risk was very low. The blood work came back first, and I did a lot of research on that particular anomaly that was very rare. I can't even remember the name of it now. How quickly I put it out of my mind!

During the pregnancy, there was a concern that my baby was a little too small—not growing in my belly and not at the right height for the number of weeks I was pregnant. So I was sent for another ultrasound in the third trimester just to be sure. It was good to have that one more chance to see the baby. He really was developing proportionately, and even though he was small, he looked just fine. I was thankful that he wasn't big. I have to say I was a bit nervous about trying to push a baby out knowing that I didn't have the largest pelvis!

I had Group B strep growing on my screening culture. I didn't want that because it meant I had to have an IV, and more than that, it meant I had to be in the hospital longer than I wanted to be.

My water broke four days before my due date. I had just gotten into bed and was feeling fine. I felt some little thing, I don't know if I'd call it a pop, but it was just a funny sensation, and then I felt the wetness. It wasn't much. It didn't actually soil the bedding, but I thought, "Hmmm." So I decided to get up and go to the bathroom to see what was going on. That's when I felt a few drops coming down my leg and I thought, "Oh! That's interesting!" When I could actually feel the dampness

If a woman has this particular bacterium as part of her normal flora, there is a slight chance of it passing to the newborn during birth. Rarely, this can cause severe infections, so some physicians give women prophylactic antibiotics to lessen the chance of infection in the baby.

and could check that in the bathroom, I noticed it was clear; there was no blood.

I had this profound realization that it was happening, that this was really *it*. I had the chills and a surge of adrenaline come over me, and I started shaking. My hands and knees started trembling. My partner had just come up to bed, so I told her what was going on. We looked at each other and we just sort of said, "*Aaaagh!*" That was at about eleven at night.

But I didn't call my doctor then. I called her at six thirty or seven in the morning. So I have to say I sort of bucked the system and purposely didn't call. I had clear fluid and the baby was moving just fine.

The person I called right away was my sister, who wanted to know when I went into labor. She got on the next airplane that morning and made it to me in time.

Unfortunately, when the water broke, it was quite a while before the contractions started. The next morning, my doctor wanted me to come in for testing to be sure the baby was safe. Normally, someone with a positive test for Group B strep must go to the hospital in the first few hours after her water breaks. She gets an IV and penicillin every four hours until the baby's born.

I knew I was going to be a long time in labor and didn't want to be in the hospital that long, so I convinced my doctor to let me stay home for about twelve hours. She did negotiate with me so that I would start on the oral antibiotics. I got the prescription and took the first dose. Then she had me come into her office for a precautionary nonstress test. And if the test had been fine, she probably would've let me go right back home.

We were put on a monitor to see that the baby's heart rate was normal and that the placenta seemed to be providing sufficient support without risk to the baby. As luck would have it, we had a decel—a decrease in the baby's heart

A nonstress test is simply using a monitor to trace the fetal heart rate while there are no contractions that would cause stress. If the heart rate shows decelerations before contractions start, this can be a cause for concern.

beat. Just one, but that one decel caused my physician to require us to go to the hospital for even more lengthy monitoring. Right off the bat, that set us up to have to work harder to get back home again.

We went to the hospital and got on the monitor, which took a little while. I had started contractions, and there was another question about the baby, so I had to stay there an extra hour. The doctor was reluctant about letting me go home at all. We got down to very specific negotiations: She would let us go home for two hours and then we had to come back, get back on the monitor, and get my first IV dose of penicillin.

That was hard because the contractions were really getting going and I was pretty uncomfortable in the car. I just wanted to go home and be home but I wasn't going to get to be home for very long. If it hadn't been hospital policy and if my physician would have been willing, I would rather not have had the penicillin, only because it tied me to the hospital more than otherwise. Even though I understand the theory of preventing transmission of Group B strep, it's statistically very unlikely that the infant would suffer any consequences. There's about one chance in four hundred that the baby would get sick from it; it's just not very common.

I tried to negotiate so that I wouldn't have to follow the hospital policy, but I wanted my physician to be comfortable, too. I knew that I wouldn't suffer any harm from the penicillin—it was just distracting because it meant I had to be at the hospital for a longer time. It was harder on Veronica than it was on me; she very much wanted to be home. By the time the contractions got started, I didn't care so much where I was—not like she did. For some reason, I was into each contraction when it came, and I just didn't want to move.

Renee did not feel a loss of power because she made a conscious and willing choice to accept the protocol.

I was getting a taste of what contractions were really like, and it was more than I bargained for, even in the beginning. How do I justify my surprise? I'd seen and helped women do this. I was disappointed that it was going to be hard for so long, but I also understood that it was what everyone goes through. I just had to buckle down, even though this was a different kind of difficulty than I'd ever dealt with before. I had to come up with a way to cope with it.

Luckily it didn't take me too long to get into a rhythm with something I could do that helped relieve each contraction. It was very simple: I just had to grab on to the shoulders of a kind person who was there to support me. I was sort of leaning forward a bit with my hands on her shoulders, and I'd breathe however I needed to breathe until each contraction passed. During almost every contraction until the final hour or two—at least every contraction where I was standing—I would do that.

My partner Veronica was wise enough to know that I needed some pressure down on my sacral bone in my lower back. So whenever there was someone available who could do that during a contraction, I would feel that pressure. It was usually Veronica, but my sister also learned how to do it. That really helped a lot, partly as a distraction, but it also seemed to lessen the pain a little bit during the contraction.

My partner was the obvious first choice for my birth team. I had some ambivalence about my mother. My mother is not one to know how to emotionally support people other than to hold somebody's hand. She has no experience in the medical field, had never seen a birth other than her own births, and couldn't even remember much about those. But she is, of all the people in my life, the person I know who loves me unconditionally. I thought, "Well, what a gift it would be if she could actually witness birth." Even if she couldn't do anything for me, I thought it would be a good thing for both of us.

It turned out that she was a great help just by standing there and letting me put my hands on her shoulders. And that really was about all she did. She didn't cook, she didn't clean, and she didn't offer any advice because she didn't know what to tell me. But she was there for me to hold on to. And the one other time in my life when I had to be in the hospital for an illness, my mother and sister were the two people who showed up for me. So it was natural that they would be the two that I would call upon.

I didn't want a lot of people involved, so I didn't include the friends that certainly could have been and were interested in being there.

Veronica had to choose somebody to be there for her as well. We had a dialogue about who that would be. A couple of our closest friends understood us well enough to do things if we needed them to without us worrying about it being a burden. We knew we could ask for their help, so we had those two friends at the birth.

I went back to the hospital because they told me I had to come back, but I would rather have stayed home a little longer. We went back on the fetal monitor for twenty minutes, and at that point the baby was no longer showing any funny heart-rate patterns. I didn't want to be stuck lying down, so the nurse got me a birthing ball that I could get up on, which I did for a while. I also went for walks in the hall, alternating between the walking and the birthing ball.

During most of the time I was in the room and on the birthing ball, I had the monitor on because it didn't bother me. I wasn't thinking about the monitor a whole lot because at that point I was tuned into getting from one contraction to the next. I turned the volume on the machine way down. One of the things that surprised me the most in retrospect was that I was not at all focused on that fetal heart-rate tracing. As a physician, I normally always watch it and tune into what's going on.

I can vaguely remember noticing a change in the heart rate, close to when the baby was born. That wasn't good, but I didn't go there, didn't engage in it, and focused on pushing. I had a feeling there was a time or two that the baby's heart rate might have been a little low, but thankfully no one made a big to-do about it. No one in the room got alarmed, and none of the doctors said a thing. And there were five doctors in the room.

The contractions seemed to come in phases, as if there were different steps or stages in my labor. The initial phase—where I was just barely dilated to maybe two or three centimeters—had a certain rhythm to it and was predictable. I knew what the next contraction was going to be like. Then when we got to five centimeters, it was still sort of predictable but harder to get through. I had to really have some help to stay focused with my breathing. It was more intense, and I wasn't so sure I was going to be able to get through it. As the contraction would build up intensity, I was afraid the peak might be more than I could handle. It seemed like it took more energy to get through each one.

At that point, I wasn't sure what physical position my body wanted to be in—if I wanted to lie down, or be on the ball, or what. Because there wasn't a relief position, there wasn't somewhere I could be during a contraction that felt better. I got frustrated. I went inside myself, and Veronica had to pull me out to stay focused on breathing. She could see that I was having trouble figuring out how to breathe. She found that if she could get me to stay focused with her that I would do better. And she had some clever ideas. She had me imagine myself on a bike ride up this big hill that we had done together, like The Little Engine that Could—I wasn't sure I could make it up there. But I did!

When I was transitioning between five and eight centimeters, I needed a dose of fentanyl because I was so tired of the escalating pain. I didn't want an epidural because I really wanted to understand what it felt like to deliver a baby. I had made a deal with myself that unless I really, really, really needed one I was not going to have an epidural. I hadn't wanted any medication, but at the same time I thought, "Hmmm… I'm not sure I'm going to be able to get through this and I don't want an epidural, so let me try something." I'm not down on myself for doing that. It helped. It didn't take the pain away, but it made it just a little less powerful at the top of the contraction. That dose lasted about an hour, and when it wore off I had another half dose.

Thank God for the spaces between the contractions because it was okay then. Between most contractions, I was able to relax. I don't know what I'd have done without that.

I don't know how long that stage was. Time warped for me. It could've been thirty minutes, and it could've been three hours; I'm not sure which.

The next thing I remember, I was lying on my side on the bed, but I was very uncomfortable, and people were telling me I was supposed to push. But I had no urge to push. All I really felt was uncomfortable. I knew that since these people knew what they were doing, that it must be true. I thought about it for about four contractions: "What am I going to do? What am I going to do?" Then I decided that I really needed to get up, even though it was going to be hard. I really needed to get up off the bed and try something else. And so I went into the bathroom and sat on the toilet.

At this point I was having a lot of rectal discomfort. It didn't feel like what I thought it was going to feel like; it didn't feel like an urge to push.

It didn't feel like hemorrhoids. It did feel a little bit like when I was really constipated once and had to spend about an hour on the toilet trying to get something out. I felt like I needed to resist it, like it was too dangerous to push into that. I was scared of that pain and couldn't imagine myself pushing into it. But I was being told by the people I trusted that I was supposed to do that.

Luckily the two helpers came into the bathroom one after the other and tried to remind me that this really was necessary, this pushing thing. And I almost needed to cry then because I was scared in a way that I hadn't been throughout the whole labor. I felt like I was up against something that was too difficult.

I don't even know what it was that Stacey said, but she was sitting right in front of me and engaging with me and

When it is time to push, the baby's head is right down by the rectum. This can cause some pain when you push, but it usually does not cause any damage. However, it can be pretty scary and the only solution is to push past the pain.

basically telling me I had to do it, but in a gentle way. In fact she was even able to tell me that she could check to see if what I was doing was working. So she coached me to just give it a try, to try to focus in on it and push to see if what I was doing was in the right place. And it seemed to be right so that gave me a little hope. Then between Veronica and Amy and Stacey I was able to get in a funny position with one knee up a little bit. It was awkward you know, sitting on the toilet. One person held a cold cloth on my head, and Veronica was behind me somewhere. There were two or three people always in there helping.

Then there was a point where there was a lull and there was nobody in the bathroom but me. I saw the clock and realized that this is it, this is my journey, and I was almost there. I knew that I just had to come up with the energy and the courage to get through this.

I really didn't believe that the baby was coming. My experience as a physician was that first babies—from the time that you are completely dilated and starting to push to the time you have the baby—take two, sometimes three hours. And I hadn't been pushing much. It seemed to me that the baby couldn't be completely descended already. That wasn't possible; that wasn't part of my paradigm of what's normal for a primagravida (first-time mother). Plus I felt nothing that I thought I was going to feel when the baby's head descended to the very edge. I thought I was going to feel the "Ring of Fire," that I would feel myself stretching, that I would know that the baby's head was there. I didn't feel that. All I felt was a pain in my butt, so I didn't believe it.

What's funny in retrospect is that I didn't check myself, because I could've felt down in that part of my body. I didn't even want to feel his head when he was actually crowning. I was so in another zone that I couldn't do it.

I was surprised that I knew when I needed to make a change. There was a certain sense of, "Okay, something needs to change." And I would change it, the position I was in or something else. Earlier, at the end of dilation, when my doctor had suggested I change positions, I wasn't ready. I had gotten into a rhythm and I was surviving that rhythm and I wasn't ready to move. Three contractions later, I was ready. I stopped and thought about what I wanted to do. I must've incorporated her request, and I thought I could do it. I would give it my best.

It's important to remain flexible about moving around during labor. Fear can get you stuck. Getting stuck in one position, no matter how comforting, can also get you stuck in your labor pattern.

I can't remember when I knew it was time to move from the bathroom, but somehow I knew to do that. Moving was scary because I knew it was the last time I was going to that bed. But it wasn't so hard to get from one place to another.

I didn't seem to have any interest in squatting. I thought about the birth ball, but I realized that it wasn't going to be helpful anymore. It was time to push. I tried lying on my side for a little bit but that didn't feel right anymore. I ended up on my back. At that point I knew I had to push, so I hunkered down. I went to bed to give it a try because I was supposed to have a baby. And I was tired of being in labor.

I had one leg that needed a little support, and I asked Amy not to let my leg move. Whenever there was something I needed or wanted,

I'd ask for it in a way that I wouldn't normally do. I would, in a matter of fact way, say, "Don't move," or "Don't change that," or "More of that pressure." I would actually just speak out and say I wanted it. Normally, I would just try to take care of it all myself or ask, "Would you mind?"

I'm guessing it was twenty minutes or a half hour after I got back to bed that he was born, but I don't know. People were talking about seeing hair, and they were getting all excited with their efforts to get me to push, so I could tell something was going on. I still didn't believe it, really. Then when the baby's head actually came out, there was a slightly different feeling—a sort of relief associated with having the big part come through. Then I realized that they weren't kidding, but I still felt disbelief. Then the baby's body came out quite easily.

It wasn't until the baby was actually on my chest and I was looking at him that I finally started to realize I had just done that. And the butt pain had gone away! Yea! That was probably the most obvious change.

So there he was, on my chest, being dried off, and I was just in awe. That moment lasted a long time. I was just staring at him in disbelief. And he was so aware that I could hardly believe that after all that, he could be awake and alert. I was just so mesmerized. And everyone else was too, and then he was taken off my belly to have some common things done, which was fine because I was getting sewn up. Everyone was gathering around and noticing how alert he was. He weighed six pounds, three ounces.

It was fun for me to see all of the people I love—my support staff—enjoying him thoroughly. And it was all right he wasn't with me because they were an extension of me and I could just watch them. It was like this circus. There were people taking pictures. There was my partner trying to get him to suckle her finger with his mouth, but because his tongue was thrusting he wasn't able to latch quite yet. She fixed his head with an osteopathic cranial treatment, and I

Common newborn baby care includes weighing and measuring, a quick examination to check his heart and lungs, and a count of fingers, toes, and other vital parts. All of this can be done without taking the baby out of the room in which he was born.

was amused. It helped me get through the painful sewing-up process. When he came back, I got to nurse, which was fun. I felt fine at that point.

Within fifteen minutes of his birth, I started feeling my brain coming back a little bit. I was able to witness what was happening inside me more. By the time we got back to the room where we were going to stay that night, I was just a tired version of myself.

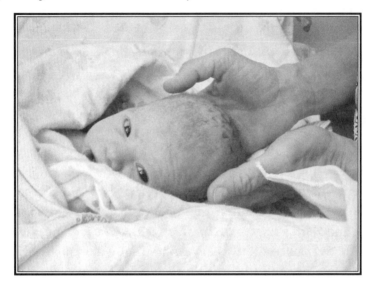

Oliver's first cranial treatment

I'm sure my baby's birth changed my professional life. Even when I was pregnant, my interactions with my pregnant patients began to change, because I was able to be with them and talk about being pregnant in a way I hadn't before. I'm able to anticipate things for people when they ask me questions about what labor's like. I guess I have—empathy is not the right word—a greater appreciation of what they're up against. Not an intellectual appreciation, but a gut appreciation, a heart appreciation, for how difficult it can be

It is important to have at least one or two people that you trust implicitly or unconditionally with you in labor and to not be shy about asking for what you need. It is important to know that it is possible, even when you think it isn't. You have to have some sort of mantra of knowing that it is possible. And it's important that you have someone with you whom you trust to be honest with you if you need to do something different.

Even before I really knew what labor was, I had a tendency to advise my patients to not get attached to their birth plan. I have yet to see someone's birth plan go exactly how she thinks it will go. I didn't make a birth plan. We always counsel people to have ideas about but not attachments to how their birth is going to be. As soon as you have an attachment to something, it's more painful when it doesn't go that way. Letting go, absolutely, is the sense of not having control over what's happening. It is powerful, and it's difficult at times.

I don't believe there is anything inherently wrong with having pain medicine. If I had needed an epidural, I would've accepted that, especially if the labor was just going nowhere and I got so tired that I didn't have the energy to push and be present for the experience of the birth. I know plenty of folks whose labors go on endlessly. They're only two centimeters dilated, and they're so exhausted that they're losing faith in everything and themselves. Without that genuine break, they can't move forward. Some would choose to have a C-section, which is definitely a riskier proposition.

It's important to be open to whatever needs to happen. A person should have a chance to be part of the process instead of being told it has to happen a certain way. I don't know that there's any wrong way to do it.

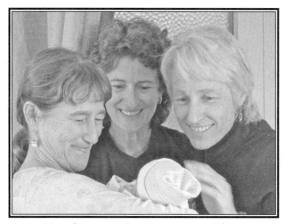

Two doctors and one aunt meet Oliver

Rainbow Wipeouts

Laura Clare and Lily

The story of Lily's birth begins before conception. Laura, a family physician with a strong spiritual faith, felt her daughter's presence long before the day of Lily's birth. Despite a series of complications and difficulties during Laura's pregnancy, her faith remained strong. She wanted a homebirth and intuitively knew it was possible, but she took the advice of all her doctors and went to the hospital instead. While there, Laura took the medical interventions in stride. She knew Lily's birth was so powerful that neither the doctor's fear nor the interventions could compromise her experience. Laura created a homebirth in the hospital in spite of everyone else's concerns.

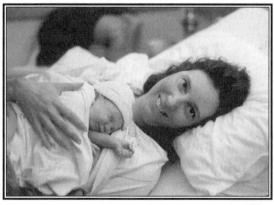

Laura and Lily

LAURA: In 1986 or '87, when I was first in medical school, it started becoming really clear that I had a strong need to have a baby. I was about thirty. I didn't think, "Oh, I just have to have a baby, any baby." It wasn't that I had to be a mommy, but there was a baby I was supposed to have. It was like this pressure that something needed to come through me.

I started looking for a daddy. After I got out of medical school, I was a family-practice resident in Santa Rosa, California. I was invited to a Halloween weekend at Sea Ranch, and one of the people there was a man who looked like pretty good daddy material. Steve and I started dating about six months later. He was totally devoted to his family and his sister, who had just been diagnosed with breast cancer. He was totally devoted to her kids. On our third date, he took me to his mother's house on Mother's Day. It was on the spur of the moment, and she had made a strawberry pie, which was my favorite. She was so delightful, she loved me, I loved her, he loved his mother, and it was all so wonderful. In retrospect I think it was all a setup and he told her to make that strawberry pie, but it worked. We decided to get married.

We made the decision in October '89 and got married in May 1990.

As soon as we had paid off the bills from getting married, I decided it was time to get pregnant. I had it all planned out. If I got pregnant in November, the baby would be born right after I got out of residency, so the timing would be perfect.

I got pregnant at the end of October, and the reason I knew I was pregnant wasn't because I had missed my period. Right before Thanksgiving, as I was driving to work early one morning, I had a vision. I had this image in my head of being in the middle of a forest in a clearing and standing there, by myself, and a voice saying to me, "No, you're not alone. We can play together and we can be together." And I knew I was pregnant.

The next day, I took the pregnancy test and it was positive. Steve and I were delighted.

The only problem was that I was a resident at the time. I was working—I was chief of surgery, actually, so I worked really long hours. Those were the eighty- to one-hundred-hour weeks. We had to take care of patients who were ill with all sorts of gross problems. The morning sickness as I sat in morning rounds while people talked about sputum and stuff like that was just beyond me. My entire surgery team was all guys. So I finally had to make a rule: They could not talk about sputum. So I got through the morning sickness, but then something else started not feeling right.

When I was about twelve weeks pregnant, I started having pain. I would try to ignore it, but it was doubled-over pain, in my lower abdomen. What it felt like more than anything was appendicitis, and that was frightening to me. And so I did what I always do: I tried to ignore it.

I ignored it for about a week and then saw my doctor. She sent me to get an ultrasound. The baby was fine, but I had these big fibroids. They were noncancerous tumors on my uterus that were growing incredibly quickly because of all the estrogen in my body. They were growing so fast they were outgrowing their blood supply, so they would die and break up inside my body, which was where the pain was coming from.

By the time I was fifteen weeks pregnant, it was affecting me so much that I passed out while I was doing a C-section. That was why I had to leave residency. I was doing a C-section with Dr. N. I had done the whole operation, we were sewing up, I handed him the needle holder, and passed out.

I had to quit. My family doctor said that she was in over her head. I went to see Dr. D, the well-known ob/gyn specialist.

My family doctor was Mary B., who had been my third-year resident. She was like a mommy when I was first learning to be a resident. (During their third year, senior residents pair up with new interns and guide them through the challenges of their first year.) She was the sweetest, kindest person I knew. She was a very soothing and comforting person. I had delivered babies with her, and she had two kids of her own. I needed a mommy—she was a mommy person.

Dr. D, who was not a mommy person, was sweet in his own way. He was a surgeon and very traditional. He examined me and was impressed with the size and number of the fibroids and the severity of the problem. He said he needed to talk with a couple of other people, and then they'd give me their plan.

A couple of days later, Steve and I went into his office. Dr. D and two other incredible surgeons planned to do the surgery. They were going to go in and remove the fibroids that were on the outside of the uterus, without disturbing the uterus or fetus. But in order to have that surgery, I had to sign consent forms. The biggest problem was that there was a really high risk of bleeding, and the only way to stop the bleeding would be to cut off the uterine arteries and take out the uterus.

I didn't even think about it. I just said, "No." Steve and Dr. D said, "Well, why not?" And I said, "Let's think about this for a minute. I have this problem. What're my chances of getting pregnant again?" And Dr. D said, "Oh no. After you have this baby you can never get pregnant again." Basically he was telling me that there was a risk that I would lose my uterus and the baby, and even if I didn't, I couldn't ever get pregnant again.

I couldn't do it. This was the Creature that Had to Be Born. So I went home to bed. And I was on pain killers during most of my pregnancy.

It hurt. It was a really bad thing. Steve took incredibly good care of me. He worked and then would come home and take care of me. He was a public health nurse at the time. He worked in Napa, and his specialty was babies and child development. He was great daddy material.

I can't say anything good about the pregnancy. I was worried because I was in bed, not working, worrying about money. At one point I thought Steve and I were going to have to move in with his parents. And I was in really bad pain, like I had appendicitis, about every ten days. If I wasn't having an attack of acute pain, I would walk around. But the pain was so frequent, and walking around made it worse. I named the fibroids. Fester was a very uncomfortable fibroid. I hated Fester.

The only time I felt good was at the YMCA. They had this swim class for pregnant people. Being in the water was wonderful because I was floating. It was great. Other than that it was pretty bad. I watched *Oprah* every day.

I was told there was a good chance that I wouldn't be able to deliver the baby naturally. One of the fibroids was down near the cervix, and it was possible that it could block the cervix.

But I personally did not anticipate any problems at all with labor and delivery. I wasn't just going to deliver the baby, I was going to deliver *me* from this terrible situation. So I was looking forward to it.

The pain was no fun, but I would have been okay except that I kept going into preterm labor. So at one point I ended up in the hospital on a terbutaline drip. Terbutaline was really icky. I cried for a day and a half. I couldn't sleep, I couldn't do anything, I just cried. The twenty-fourth through twenty-sixth weeks were the hardest. I knew about preterm babies and intensive care nurseries, and it was the last thing in the world I wanted for my baby. They could be born and they could be saved, but it wasn't a good thing.

Through all of it, the baby was incredibly healthy. She was growing just like she was supposed to. Nothing was wrong with her.

I would've loved to deliver at home, but it was never an option. I delivered babies, I knew the midwives, and I totally trusted them. There were good midwives in Sonoma County, but there was a little bit of back-and-forth about delivering in Healdsburg because the midwives did not deliver in our little hospital. They followed a protocol that required them to practice within twenty minutes of a tertiary care nursery. I knew all about them.

These midwives were incredible. They had these setups where they could handle anything. And the big hospital wasn't that much fun for me. It was my workplace. It was yucky. So I would've loved to deliver at home or locally, but it was never an option. I fell into all the risk categories, so the midwives wouldn't see me as a patient.

I figured I had the next best thing: I had a family doctor who had taught me how to do family-centered birthing and was a staunch supporter of it. We were going to do this in a hospital that supported family-centered birthing, and it was going to be the next best thing to birthing at home.

In family-centered birthing, the purpose of the birth is to deliver not only a healthy baby, but a happy baby. The family gets to call the shots. The delivery of the baby was the defining moment of the family, any family. And so having the family being the center of the delivery instead of accessories to the vagina was the goal of the birth experience. Oh God, I believed it so strongly!

I was in preterm labor from twenty-four to twenty-eight weeks. In the first week in May, when I was close to twenty-eight weeks pregnant, Steve gave me injections to help mature the baby's lungs. We thought she was going to be delivered quite early. She was due August 1st.

But the strangest thing happened. Once we got into the third trimester, the fibroids pretty much settled down. They settled down, and I was just one big pregnant lady. I looked like I was carrying twins, but it was okay. I didn't hurt as much anymore, I wasn't having the contractions anymore, and it was summertime. Every day I ate a whole watermelon and waddled all around town.

I was having ultrasounds all the time at that point so that we could see if the fibroid that was close to my cervix was in the way. I had steadfastly refused to allow them to tell me the sex of the baby. But looking at the ultrasound on July 11th, I knew she was a little girl. She was beautiful, and I was so happy. It was a solar eclipse that day, which was magical. I thought, "Everything's going to be okay. I'm having a girl, and I'm not sick anymore." I was just totally accepting this. And of course I was really looking forward to labor.

On July 15th I woke up in the morning and went out to the garden and was squatting, you know, like in *The Good Earth*. I was digging in the garden and all this water ran down my legs. I clearly was not peeing, which was always a possibility at that point. My water had broken. I was amazed. "Oh man, this stuff really happens!"

I called my family doctor, Mary, and she said, "Great, just stay in touch and let me know if anything else happens." I wasn't having any contractions. I think I called my friend Stacey before I called Steve. He was at work, and I wasn't sure it was for real. Stacey said, "I'll be right up," and she was there in half an hour. When she walked in the house, I was there on my hands and knees on the floor and I was just rocking back and forth. I said, "You know, I haven't had any contractions, and I'm not really in labor." And she started laughing really loud. She said, "Look, you're on the floor, on your hands and knees, rocking. You're in labor, okay?"

But it didn't hurt. I mean, I had sensations, and I don't know if it didn't hurt because of the pain I'd already gone through, or if my body was just doing what it was supposed to do. It really didn't feel like pain.

There was something bigger than my will or ego that was taking over. I had the sensation that the baby was calling the shots. I was having contractions. They were Braxton Hicks contractions; I could feel everything tighten up, but it didn't hurt. When the contraction would go away, there was this opening feeling inside of me. The reason I was rocking was just to stay as loose as possible.

I remember not having any Kotex or pads, and I thought I needed them. Stacey and I walked to the store, which was two blocks away, bought pads, and came back. Somewhere in there was when we called Steve.

Steve went into daddy hysteria at work, causing the women at work to break out in gales of laughter. He was pretty hysterical by the time he got to the house. Stacey and I were just sitting there, gossiping. He said, "Hey! Why aren't we boiling water and stuff?"

I just don't remember all that happened between ten o'clock when my water broke and around four in the afternoon when Mary said, "You need to go ahead and go to the hospital." I said, "I'm not having contractions!" and she said, "Why don't you go ahead and go to the hospital so we can figure out where you're at and what's going to happen."

I didn't want to go to the hospital. I just felt that this was such a good thing, and everything was going to be okay. I could've just stayed on my hands and knees and had that baby there in my house. That's what I wanted to do.

But I did go to the hospital because I had to. Nobody thought it was safe for me to have that baby at home.

Luckily the nice big birthing room was open. It was such a beautiful day. I was thinking, "God I don't really need to be here. I'm not having contractions." I started running up and down the four flights of stairs to see if I could make the contractions happen.

Mary B came after work; it was after five. They must've put monitors on me because I have a photograph of me lying on the bed with my big old belly sticking straight up. I didn't have the monitors on in the picture but the only reason I would've been lying down on the bed is because they were doing intake kind of things. I was just laughing and smiling. Steve and Stacey were there. Those are the only people I wanted there. I had done plenty of deliveries by that time, and one of the things I could never understand was why people would have a long list of guests they wanted at the delivery.

I was completely effaced but not dilated at all. Not even a fingertip. I think Mary was waiting a long time before she checked me because she didn't want to start that clock. Once the cervix is checked after the waters break, the baby must be delivered within twelve hours or the risk of infection becomes a concern. I know Mary, and she was nervous. She was worried about this not being the easiest delivery. But her nervousness didn't bother me. I really believed that this was a process that was going to go however it went despite the doctor being nervous—and in her nervousness probably wanting to be more interventionist than she would normally have been.

She decided we needed to start Pitocin at seven in the evening. I didn't care one way or the other. The thing is, Stacey really questioned

Mary, asking "Why are we doing this?" and Mary's response was, "We don't know if she's going to have a normal contraction pattern or a normal labor." And who knows why? We didn't need the Pitocin, but she was worried.

I had this contraction—boom! It hit and I breathed through it. No one was paying any attention to me; they were doing other things. When I came out of it, I looked around and said very loudly, "Well, you gotta watch what you wish for." Because I had been wanting these contractions to start, and *man*, did they start.

I'd start to feel the tightening. It was just a little tinge of the feeling, and then all of a sudden this huge pain would start right under my ribs and run all the way down my body. Steve was right there, and he was going to breathe with me. They were coming pretty quick, like every three or four minutes. When it started, it started.

I had gone through prepared childbirth classes and had already figured out that I was going to pretend like I was surfing, you know, up and over the waves. It was going to be great. I started doing my visualization of up and over the waves and damn, I ended up being in the waves. I ended up wiping out—head over heels. And at one point I realized that I was inside my own womb. The wave would come up, curl down over me, and come crashing down on me. I was inside this watery place. I was inside the womb, and the pain was my whole world, just for those few minutes.

When Pitocin brings on contractions like these, the nurse usually turns the IV off to avoid overstimulating labor. The body then takes over naturally.

I was breathing like I was supposed to. I wasn't aware of the room or anybody talking because I was hallucinating. The thing was, inside that womb it wasn't dark. It was rainbow colors. There was color washing over me. I was spinning head over heels in a wave in the water. Then it would start to let up and I would be back in the labor room again.

I was laboring sitting up. I had the bed in the folded sit-up position. I was not on my feet squatting. Steve was wiping my face with cool washcloths and giving me ice, and Stacey was helping me breathe.

There was a labor nurse, Dani. She was a really short woman, not someone we were familiar with. She was salt of the earth, talking to me and saying, "Okay, now this is what's going to happen." And then it would happen. She was doing Shiatsu massage on pressure points on my ankles. It felt so good. She said, "This helps you to open up. As long as you're going to have contractions like this, they might as well be doing something." The Pitocin seemed totally superfluous to me.

This started at seven fifteen and got more and more intense. I started getting pretty wild. I wasn't standing up, but I was all over the place on the bed and I can remember saying those silly words women say, like "I can't do this" and "I want to go home now." I was thinking, "I have to have a C-section," but I didn't say that out loud. Even I knew that was silly, but now I knew, "Oh that's why all those women say that." It was impossible to imagine going through that experience and surviving it.

But at the same time I knew that it was going to be great, and the only way through it was straight through it. At one point Steve was in my face saying, "You're doing so well!" I looked up at him sort of cross-eyed and he looked totally happy. I was so pissed. I couldn't believe that he could be that happy when I was obviously dying. I grabbed his ponytail and I yanked it really hard until he got right in my face and I said, "You motherfucker, wipe that smile off your face!" Which he laughed at.

I sensed something was happening because I was getting violent. Both Stacey and Dani decided that I needed to be checked again. Mary came in and checked me, and I remember the look on her face. It was like, "This can not be. This can not be." It had been less than two hours. It was nine o'clock, and I was completely dilated. In less than two hours I went from totally closed to completely dilated, which probably accounts for the hallucinations.

There was jubilation in the room, and everyone was so happy for me. I was still hallucinating.

This was supposed to be good because now I could push, and I always told my patients that they were going to feel better when they could push. That was of course after they had gone through eight hours of labor. So Mary said, "Why don't you get up and see if you can pee, and then you can try pushing." Good idea. Thank you. So I got up and I had this stupid IV pole with me. I was tethered to it. So I took a few steps over to the toilet and peed, and then, "Oh my God, another one's coming!" How was I going to handle this sitting on the toilet? I was going to start hallucinating. There was a voice that said, "Push."

I tried pushing, and it felt like my rectum was being torn in two, and I got scared. That's really the only time I got scared. I stood up with the IV pole and looked at everybody. They were very happy, and I decided that they were all in on it. They were all trying to kill me, and especially that baby. I had to get out of there. I took the IV pole and started running. I couldn't get very far, but I was running around the room. People started yelling at me and Steve got me back in bed. I don't think I'm making this up, because how could I make that up? I was scared.

I was lying on my left side. Stacey was holding my right leg up and I was grabbing onto my left leg, pulling my knee up onto my chest. Steve said, "You have to do this." I said, "I know." And so I pushed. During the next contraction, I took a big breath, pushed, let out the sound that my sister calls the "dying elephant" sound—she's had five kids—and pushed right through that pain. I mean, really truly, there was something very big happening in my body, but I pushed right through it.

Steve was really happy. He was jumping up and down and saying, "Yes! Yes!" because he thought that noise was so good. I had one more dying-elephant-sound contraction, and the baby was crowning. I could reach down and feel her head, and Stacey was deliriously happy. She was encouraging me.

Mary said, "I think you're going to rip. I'm going to cut an episiotomy." And I didn't even care. I mean, I literally did not feel her cutting it. As it turned out, it was a pretty good, controlled delivery. She told me when to push and when to stop, and that's what I did. Once we got back in bed after running around the room, it took half a dozen pushes to deliver that baby. It was the most amazing feeling.

I felt like I had just created the whole world. It was just incredible, that spiritual feeling of oneness that is so elusive—the feeling of oneness with all of creation. Like I was the Goddess and I had just created the World. And at the same time there was a little part of my mind that was thinking, "Wow this is pretty weird! You have a baby now."

So Mary delivered her and put her on my belly. Lily started wailing. I don't remember any of the "take the baby over to the incubator" thing. I don't think I let go of her! She was crying, and Steve helped me pick her up and move her up to my breast, but she didn't nurse. She had no interest. I remember her just wailing for ten minutes or so. I was pretty worn out. It just got really quiet as Mary was sewing me up. She was apologizing, "I'm sorry; I didn't need to cut this episiotomy. I'm so sorry."

What advice would I give Lily? Lily's so stubborn, what can I tell her?

The only way to have a baby is to surrender, let go, and let the baby do what the baby has to do. Let your body support the baby. It's not just during labor. I think it's a frame of mind that you need to have from the beginning.

It's good to read and know all about what it's like to have a baby, and to go to childbirth classes. But I have a real bias against birth plans because I have a bias against thinking you have control over this. Not to say that you don't make the best choices you can, like having Mary as my doctor because she was a mother and supported the family birthing that I wanted to do. And I knew that I wanted Stacey there with me.

I had a feeling that birth was bigger than all the interventions. Bigger than Pitocin. If I had had a birth plan that said, "I don't believe in Pitocin; never ever use it," I would've been fighting that instead of doing what I needed to do which was to let go and let the baby come. And that was going to happen, Pitocin or no Pitocin.

The letting-go thing is very, very important. Having Lily was the most spiritual thing I've ever done. It was a power much greater than me running the show. I trusted that it was going to be okay. I'm happy that I trusted that because that's how I got to have that feeling that I had just created the whole world—that moment of unity with all.

I'm really happy that Lily's first breaths were in that kind of energy, the spiritual energy that was all around her when she was born.

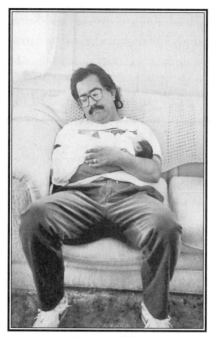

Steve and Lily

THIRD TIME'S THE CHARM

CHRISSY AND ANAEL

Chrissy is more comfortable telling stories with her photographs, and she is quite good at her craft. So I wrote her story for her, and she still gives me wonderful photos of her daughter as Anael grows to be a beautiful young girl.

※

Chrissy was pregnant. It was bad timing. She had just moved to the area and had a dream job working as a photographer for the local newspaper. Her boyfriend was serious, but she wasn't ready to marry him, and they were certainly not ready to settle down and have a family. Things were moving way too fast.

We discussed her options. After talking about abortion, adoption, and motherhood, she left to consider the situation and to discuss it with David. She was going to call me in another week or so with their plan. But before the week was out, Mother Nature took over.

Chrissy had a miscarriage. It was not painful, she had no complications, and she was philosophical about it. She saw that this miscarriage had taken the decision out of her hands and given her the freedom to plan her family with more conscious intent.

About a year later, Chrissy came back to see me. She was again pregnant and this time she was ecstatic. She and David were solid, the job was going well, and this pregnancy was a blessing. We started her prenatal care.

The pregnancy was going well until two days short of her twentieth week. In the middle of the night, without warning, her water broke. She and David spent hours that night in the emergency room and were told there was nothing anyone could do; they should go home and call me in

137

the morning. It had been almost a month since her last prenatal visit and she was due to see me anyway. So when David called that next morning, I asked them to come into the office. When they walked in the door, I knew. I could see it in her face and in her body, and I could feel it in the energy. Chrissy was having this baby and she was having it today. She was terrified about what was happening to her, how she felt, and that her much-wanted baby would not survive. When I checked her, she was already four centimeters dilated. It was too late to do anything other than deliver this child.

We couldn't deliver the baby in my office, so I got on the phone to find a place that would be supportive. This family could not be on the regular labor and delivery ward—that would have been unnecessarily cruel, forcing them to hear the first cries of healthy newborns. I called a hospital that I knew had a compassionate staff that could manage a situation like this, but they didn't have a single bed available that day. I tried the small hospital near my office and asked if they could accommodate this family's needs. They had no facilities for delivering babies, but they were willing to do what they could. Because they had no nursing staff trained in obstetrics, I cancelled my appointments for the day and went with David and Chrissy to the hospital. We spent that day together delivering their baby boy.

Obadella did not survive. We knew he wouldn't. We just had to get through this awful day together with as much grace and compassion as we could. The nurses were wonderful, bringing me everything I asked for after searching through the storeroom for instruments and supplies. Some of those instruments hadn't been used for twenty years. The staff did everything they could to support this little family in their grief. The supervisor went home in the middle of her day and found a small basket shaped like a heart; she lined it with a soft yellow baby blanket and when Obadella was born, we tucked him in. David and Chrissy spent some time with their baby, bonding and grieving simultaneously before they let him go. The birthing energy rarely feels as sad as it did that day.

Chrissy grieved for many months. She took time off work. Taking photographs for the newspaper no longer seemed important. The dream job had become an unwanted responsibility that overwhelmed her. For many months, nothing seemed important. Slowly she recovered her joy in life, sense of humor, and optimism. But the fear of another loss remained. She knew that only a successful pregnancy would heal that wound.

Chrissy and David decided to get married. On a beautiful sunny spring day, they had a ceremony in a huge ocean-side garden full of blossoms, cooled by the breezes coming off of the northern California Pacific Ocean. It was a huge wedding with all their friends and family to bless them. David, accomplished on the bagpipes, was dressed in full kilt regalia and serenaded his bride during the reception. It was a day of celebration, new hope, and healing.

And then Chrissy got pregnant again. We talked about her fears and discussed how this pregnancy would be managed differently. Because of the timing and the way Obadella came, I was suspicious that Chrissy might have an "incompetent cervix," which is a cervix that spontaneously shortens and dilates halfway through the pregnancy instead of holding tight until a full forty weeks has passed. We agreed that we didn't like the term, and decided to call it an "overeager cervix" or even an "overenthusiastic cervix" —more positive terms that wouldn't make her feel like a failure.

Although we needed the specialist for the stitching on her cervix, we did not need him for the whole pregnancy. Mary wanted a natural delivery, so we continued to work together on the normal parts of her pregnancy while the obstetrician managed the abnormal cervix for us.

During the first months of her pregnancy, we did sonograms of her cervix every week. When we noticed that it was shortening, I called my friendly obstetrician and he put a few stitches in the cervix to hold it closed. This was a procedure requiring the skills and instruments of a specialist, beyond the scope of my own practice. He put her on bed rest and she was down for the rest of her pregnancy, allowed up off the couch only to go to the bathroom, get something out of the fridge, or come to her regular prenatal appointments. It was going to be a long pregnancy, but the fear was lessening each week. She felt safer with the knowledge that we were doing everything we could to manage this pregnancy and avoid another loss. Each week that passed was a cause for celebration.

Chrissy set up court in her living room. Her laptop computer, books, projects and friends surrounded her for the next six months. She had a baby shower with a Red Tent theme because at the time, we were all reading *The Red Tent*, a book that celebrates womanhood and community. All the lamps were covered with red scarves, and the house was full of women, good food, laughter, and baby gifts. She was glowing. She was not afraid.

At about thirty-eight weeks, the stitches were taken out of her cervix and the obstetrician signed off on her case. We were all ready to go to the hospital any moment now that her cervix was free. And of course, nothing happened. That cervix seemed to have a mind of its own and now that it was time, it refused to dilate. Chrissy spent the last three weeks of her pregnancy waiting anxiously, like most other pregnant women. She was glad to have this time and used it to get her strength back. After lying around for months, her legs felt weak, and she needed to learn to be active again. She was in training to be a new mother.

One full week after the due date, labor finally started. She and David planned to stay at home as long as possible during the early part of labor and go to the hospital only when it became necessary. Although Chrissy had been through labor before, she knew it would be more intense this time around with a bigger baby to deliver. She also had every intention of photographing her baby's birth as it happened. When I laughed at her optimism, she agreed that she might be too busy to take photos while she pushed her baby out, but she was going to have the camera at her side anyway, just in case.

The labor for Anael was as normal as it gets. Chrissy worked hard and asked for no medications, and David supported her throughout. It was as if all their fear had been used up during the last year and they had been burned clean by that process. All that was left was their joy when they brought a healthy baby into their family.

As sometimes happens after a normal labor, there were problems during the actual delivery. Chrissy was still hoping to take photographs as she delivered her child, but after the head was delivered, the shoulders would not come. Shoulders can take as much effort and energy to deliver as the baby's head, and this was a classic case of shoulder dystocia. I was doing everything I knew to get that baby out. Chrissy was pushing with all her might. She had delivered while lying on her back, so her knees were up by her shoulders making her pelvis as wide as possible. The nurse was putting pressure in just the right place to encourage movement. I was working to rotate the baby's body, first one way and then the other, trying to get that shoulder under and past the pubic bone.

The seconds passing seemed like hours. We knew we would need to give this baby some resuscitation when we got her out. Just as I was ready to ask Chrissy to flip over onto her hands and knees, Anael's shoulder slipped out and I was able to deliver her up onto her mother's belly.

Anael was limp, pale, and not making any effort to breathe or move. We quickly cut her cord and moved her over to our resuscitation table, right there in the room where she was delivered. A quick assessment verified that her heart was beating well, so we got the oxygen out and started stimulating her to breathe on her own. Again, the seconds seemed like hours, but in my heart I knew Anael was going to be all right. We had not come this far only to lose her. She just needed some help to start up. David was holding his baby's hand, pulling her into life with his love and his will; Chrissy had finally grabbed her camera. She was holding the camera in her hand, but covering her eyes with the other hand; she couldn't bear to watch while she anxiously waited for her daughter's first cry. The seconds ticked by.

The miracle of Anael came first in the pinking of her face and body, then in little grunts as she tried out her lungs. Slowly she began to breathe on her own and return her father's pressure on her hand. Her eyes opened and we knew we had her. That first cry came and the whole room lit up with relief, joy, and gratitude.

Anael Zaia, all eight pounds, nine ounces of this much-wanted and long-awaited

The quickest way out of a shoulder dystocia is to have the woman flip over onto her hands and knees—the Gaskin Maneuver. This maneuver releases the stuck shoulder and the baby slides right out. It can be daunting to move when you are in that position, but it is important to know that you can, especially if you do not have a deep epidural preventing you from feeling your own legs.

The level of resuscitation that Anael needed could also have been provided by an experienced midwife in a homebirth. Although we had a nice warming table with suction and oxygen attached, these supplies should also be part of a midwife's kit.

baby girl was here to stay. The cameras started clicking. In that moment, a family was born.

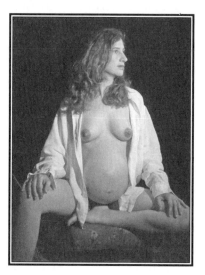

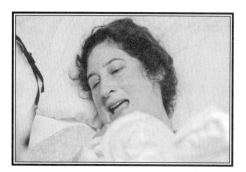

Just as I was ready to ask Chrissy to flip over, Anael's shoulder slipped out, and I was able to flip her up onto her mother's belly.

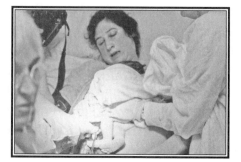

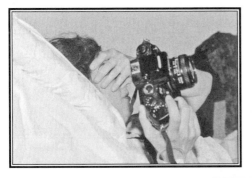

Chrissy had finally grabbed her camera. She was holding the camera in her hand, but covering her eyes with the other hand; she couldn't bear to watch while she anxiously waited for her daughter's first cry.

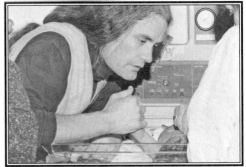

We had not come this far only to lose Anael. She just needed some help to start up. David was holding his baby's hand, pulling her into life with his love and his will.

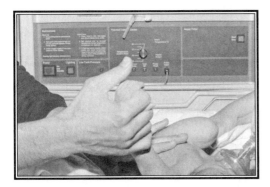

The miracle of Anael came first in the pinking of her face and body…

That first cry came and the whole room lit up with relief, joy, and gratitude.

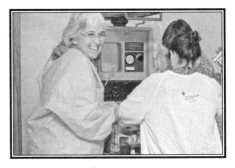

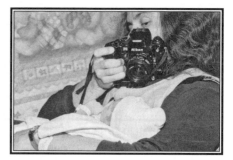

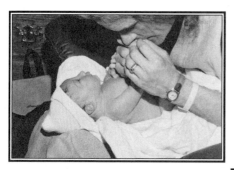

The cameras started clicking.
In that moment, a family was born.

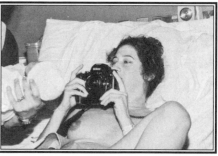

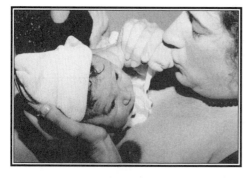

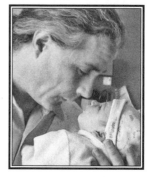

INTUITIVE, INTROSPECTIVE, INSPIRATIONAL

LENNIE AND ZAN CAYLI AND EYAN

Lennie is an accomplished actress, producer, and director. She is an acting coach with rare talent, and she raises her children in an environment rich with art and creativity.

I first met Lennie when I was a resident physician in training. I had been assigned to an evening clinic for "high-risk" pregnancies. These were women who, for whatever reason, needed special care. In Lennie's case, she had just moved from New York City, was without a doctor seven months into her pregnancy, had high blood pressure, and was an older mother. She was a very large woman who carried a lot of extra weight with the pregnancy.

I was not enthusiastic about my job that night. I didn't like working nights and would rather have been home with my own two children. I had no ongoing relationship with any of these women. I was simply doing high-risk intake and referring patients on to other providers for the rest of their pregnancies. But Lennie brightened my night. Here was this very large woman—huge in pregnancy—with the personality of an actor. All those pregnant emotions were right out there, and I knew that what I saw was a real, no-nonsense, honest woman. She had bright red hair, freckles that covered every surface of her body, and a smile that warmed my heart. When I realized her due date was the same as my own birthday, I invited her into my personal clinic and agreed to be there to deliver her baby.

Lennie doesn't do anything halfway, and her life is never boring. Between a car accident and her high blood pressure, she packed nine months of drama into the last three months of this pregnancy. Her story makes clear why I chose to be a family doctor instead of a midwife. I needed a broad range of medical skills to help Lennie through those last months, and because I had those skills I was able to advocate and care for her no matter what happened.

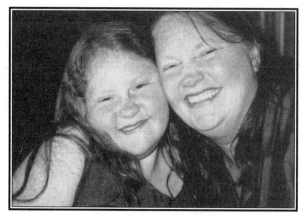

Zan Cayli and Lennie

LENNIE: I was thirty-nine when Zan came along. We had just moved to California from New York and I was seven months pregnant, had high blood pressure, and needed to find a doctor soon. I was having difficulty giving my one-year-old, Edienna, what she needed. Ben was traveling back and forth to L.A. for acting jobs. I found a doctor within the first week of arriving in California, and that was a good thing!

When I was eight months pregnant with Zan, I got in an automobile accident.

It was a beautiful September day. I was sitting in the front seat of my husband's car, and he was driving. My mother was in the back seat. We were on our way home from a garage sale, getting ready to go to my baby shower. Some kid, who was probably nineteen or twenty years old, made a left turn in front of us. Bad judgment on his part. We hit him directly in the side of his car. Ben slammed on the brakes, and my mother said, "Oh my God!" and reached up and grabbed my shoulder. When I saw it was going to happen, I completely relaxed and went inside with the baby. I closed my eyes and leaned back in my seat and just went right inside and got completely relaxed. I had my seat belt on. I had just seen a special on TV about how best to wear seat belts when you are pregnant: it should be across the wide part of the belly, rather than the lower part of the body. I was proud of myself for having worn it properly.

The car was totaled. The entire front of the car was shoved in so the dash hit my knee, shattering my kneecap. The first thing I did when the car stopped was to communicate with the baby by massaging my uterus. My whole body was in panic mode with adrenalin shooting through me, and my belly was as hard as a rock. I just kept thinking about my high blood pressure, so I kept breathing deeply and praying. I was really talking to the baby. I wanted to feel movement. I didn't feel it move but kept saying, "Okay, please baby, you're okay. You're safe. It's okay." I tried to be calming because I knew there was panic inside there too.

Ben was really angry. He first came to see how I was, and then he went toward the other car. He was screaming at the guy and I got a little frightened about that. Then the next moment Ben was next to me and I said, "I need you to stop and be quiet and help me. And let's not be panicked. That's what I need right now." And he changed instantly. My knee didn't hurt but I did feel a dent there. I knew something was wrong but at each turn, when I was checking myself out, the most important thing was the baby again. I couldn't focus on anything else.

Babies are well protected inside the uterus and inside the amniotic sac, floating in their water. Nature is well designed to protect our babies from most traumas. But they do feel our emotions and our stress hormones, so Lennie was right to calm herself for the sake of the baby.

An ambulance came and took my mother and me to the hospital. She was there to hold my hand and remind me that Baby was going to be fine. I remember them taking my blood pressure and it was really sky high. I kept working toward calming down. The paramedics were really nice about it, and I don't really remember much pain. I think I even felt a little movement from the baby during the ambulance ride.

DR. KERR: I was working in the hospital that day, doing rounds and having a regular, crazy, busy resident day. I was paged and informed that one of my pregnant patients had just been brought into the ER; she'd been in a car accident. I ran to the ER immediately, not sure what I was going to find. It was a relief to see Lennie intact, not bleeding, and mostly just scared out of her wits. My first order of business was to calm everyone down.

A doctor who is also your trusted advocate can provide a safe place for you in the hospital.

LENNIE: The first time I cried was when Stacey met me in the ER. When she showed up, I felt really sure that it was going to be okay. I could let go some. It allowed me to feel what I needed to feel for myself, not just the baby. And that is when I started feeling contractions. Ben couldn't be there, my mother was being seen in another room, and it was really important to have my doctor there stroking my hand and telling me, "It's okay. If we have a baby today it will be fine. Don't you worry about it." I felt nurtured and safe.

The sonogram told us that the baby was fine and the placenta was intact. They x-rayed my knee, found it to be in three pieces, and admitted me to the hospital to monitor the baby and figure out how to fix my knee. But they didn't know where to put me. Should I be on the maternity ward? Should I be downstairs in the orthopedic ward? Nobody wanted to handle the other ward's issue. I needed surgery on my knee, but the first anesthesiologist who came in was freaked. He was scared that the baby was going to come and he did not want to deal with that.

The sense I got was that I frightened people and they didn't know where I belonged. Finally, a day or two later (which I spent up on the maternity ward), we got an anesthesiologist who would give me an epidural. If the baby decided to come while they were fixing my knee, we would just move that stuff out of the way and the baby would be delivered. I was still having little contractions. I think they continued for two or three days after the accident. We didn't use any medicine to stop them, and finally they did stop on their own.

DR. KERR: Lennie had shattered her kneecap and the three separate pieces needed to be wired together during her surgery. We had her hooked up to a fetal monitor the whole time so we would know if the baby was stressed or if labor was starting. I never doubted that this baby would wait for her own time. Lennie's kids want their own spotlight whenever possible. The orthopedic surgeon and I worked for several hours on Lennie's leg and there were no complications.

LENNIE: It was after the surgery that I really felt the pain from my knee. It was just incredible pressure, like an elephant standing on it. It was unbearable; I just lost it. Now I was on the orthopedic ward, and nobody wanted to deal with me. They didn't know what to do with me and the baby. Finally a doctor came down from the obstetric area and talked to me. She said, "You have got to shape up and stop this. You have got to consider the baby. You are getting all upset, and you have to find a way to manage the pain because you're just getting your blood pressure up and getting yourself all in a tizzy. So whatever it is you need to do, just do it because this is not good for you or the baby."

Lennie is still grateful to this doctor who visited her that night. She needed a reality check, and the directness of this doctor's message got through to her. She was getting pain medication, but the anxiety was overwhelming. She could not let her emotions take over.

I came out of surgery with a long leg cast, which was bright, Day-Glo pink. That hot pink cast clashed with everything—my red hair and everything else about me. I had to lie flat in bed the entire time I had it on, about eight weeks. It was not what I expected at all. It was a particularly hot October. I was staying at my sister's home, and two-year-old Edie would not come near the special hospital bed so I couldn't spend any time with her at all. Ben was hauling bedpans because I couldn't even get out of bed or clean myself. I am a very big woman, too. I was just pretty depressed.

I went through a couple of false labors before I finally went into the real thing.

The last weeks of pregnancy are often the hardest, especially when there are special circumstances. This is where we get to learn the patience and tolerance it takes to raise children.

When I knew I was really in labor, I was elated. I wanted to meet my baby and know that she was okay. I called the hospital and they were pretty busy; they told me to take a shower and have something to eat, then to come in. I took a sponge bath (no showers with a cast!) and went for tacos, then was admitted to the hospital at seven in the evening. I forgot about the problem with my leg and everything else because of the anticipation of the beauty of birth.

Laboring was interesting because I could not move around. I had a friend there who had three children herself and she was surprised, saying, "I can't believe that you're having contractions because you just get so quiet." I just have a way of looking inside. All my energy just goes and looks inside and sees what's going on. I would breathe and feel and go in and examine once again. And that was wonderful for awhile. Then, the last part of my labor was really, really intense. I had really intense pain. It was not in the back; it was in the front part of my body. I remember pushing on the cast with my hands. I'd beat on the cast with my hands. We weren't sure that the baby was going to be born that night or the early morning because I wasn't quite dilated. It was going slow for the first four or five hours. But I didn't take any Pitocin or pain medicine.

The next thing I remember was Stacey breaking my water to speed things up. That's when I started screaming and yelling. I was an absolute mess.

DR. KERR: I broke her membranes because she was not making progress as a result of all of her hard work, and rupturing the bag of waters will often allow the baby's head to press down on the cervix. This can help dilate the cervix and intensify the labor, speeding things up without using medications. I always discuss this with the mother before I do it. We discuss the pros and cons, and I make sure I have her full agreement. Lennie agreed, but then thought better of it when her contractions immediately came on so strong. By then it was too late.

LENNIE: I felt that I had to apologize for my behavior. I remember feeling sorry that I was being so loud. I remember saying, "Sorry, sorry, I'm sorry!" and "No, no, no, no," and everybody kept saying, "Say yes Lennie. Say yes. Open up, come on, open up." Finally I quit caring and started really screaming and being vocal. I think that really helped because it is an expression of energy and allows it to be freed.

When you let go of all the feelings with a sigh or scream, you release it and you can go on to the next moment. If you're hanging on to it, it's more intense and it can't do its work. You hold it still because you think it's going to make it better and it doesn't. That's what happened to me earlier: A nurse watched me through a contraction and said, "You know, don't go inside. Stay with Ben. Watch him and look in his eyes and let him help you through it." It was more intense when I was going inside and examining all the feelings rather than having an outside focus.

I have managed my way through each of my births by determining for myself what's going on. I don't know if my determinations are accurate or not, but it is what I do. When my water was broken, I felt the baby's head pressing right on my cervix. I was pissed at the doctor for making it be so intense so suddenly. My blood pressure was up again. I could feel myself stretching and every time I stretched, there was extreme pressure from the baby's head, a deep burning inside my body. When I asked for drugs, I was too far along to get them.

When I knew it was coming, any second, I knew there wouldn't be any pushing. When I open up, the baby's head is just right there. It was the same for my mother. I was being told to pant so they could get me to the special delivery room. We had decided to go there because of the cast complication. We had to get a huge plastic bag over the cast to protect it.

We had experimented through the night with different positions, holding my leg up and finding the way that I was the most open. There was a nurse there to hold the leg, a woman who was filming the birth for me, my own doctor, and an obstetric specialist in case we got in trouble.

So finally we were all there, and the first thing Stacey said was, "She has your hair! Curly red hair!" and the other doctor said, "Push, come on Lennie, push, push, push!" I didn't feel like I was having trouble pushing. I remember him saying, "Don't stop. Let's get it out, get it out altogether, at once. No breathing in between because we don't want the shoulder to retract."

So she came out. It was five in the morning. I was asking, "How is she? Is she okay?" because I was still worried about the accident. They had to take her and suction her because there was a little meconium in the fluid. Ben went right to her when that was happening. I was having strong contractions still so that I could deliver the placenta. I remember being pissed and surprised that they were so intense after she was out.

I tore my cervix, and we had to fix that.

I remember her working so hard to focus and making cat sounds. Sweet, sweet sounds. She was big—eight pounds, five ounces—and I could not wait to have her in my arms. What a great joy it was to look at her, tell her how much I loved her, and have her really look at and focus on me. We felt an instant connection. She nursed within fifteen minutes, and since I still couldn't get out of bed, she and I were very, very close. Zan took to nursing right away. She stayed in my arms 100 percent of the time, and it was lovely.

I had planned to have my tubes tied after Zan was born, so we set up a time on the day after the birth to do that. I came in, they got me on the operating table, and they tried to start an IV for me. If I was stuck once, I was stuck thirty times. I mean every single person in that hospital was called to come in and try. They looked at my toes, they looked at my entire body, and there was no vein to be found. Finally Stacey came in and looked at me and said, "About our only alternative is a jugular vein in your neck. This doesn't seem like the right thing to do. There is something more powerful going on here. I don't know, it's up to you, and you do have these options. But I've got to tell you, I don't think it's going to happen today." And I had that feeling too, big time. So I said, "Okay, never mind," got off the operating table, and went home.

And that is why I have another tale to tell.

Occasionally the cervix will tear during a delivery but this is not dangerous. (The midwife or doctor will simply repair it to prevent complications from any bleeding.) But she was beautiful. She was not very loud—a quiet girl with a little twisted mouth. She's still got a beautiful twisted mouth.

DR. KERR: By the time Eyan was born three years later, I was no longer a resident and was in private practice across town from the hospital. In the middle of the night, I could get to the hospital in ten minutes or less, but in the middle of the afternoon it could take twenty minutes or more to negotiate my way through traffic. I always asked the nurses to take that into account when deciding when to call me in. Unlike midwives, doctors keep their regular appointments while women are in labor. We do very little labor sitting and rely on the nurses to keep us informed and tell us when it's time to come catch the baby.

Early in my career, I tried to labor sit. To my surprise, it did not help. As a matter of fact, it seemed to slow things down to have the doctor "hovering." After several births, I let the women labor on their own with their families to support them and the nurses to monitor Mother Nature's needs. These births went more quickly. Most mothers wanted me there when the delivery was close, but they were content with their doulas, sisters, husbands, and mothers sitting with them through the earlier parts of labor.

I enjoyed delivering at the hospital where I had trained. I knew the nurses and trusted them. They knew me and trusted my skill and judgment. This good working relationship helped me deliver babies the way I felt was best: with minimal intervention and good communication with the family. And I made a promise to all the parents—one that was becoming increasingly rare in the medical community: I personally would be there to deliver the baby. I would schedule nothing more important than the arrival of their child. They could count on it.

Occasionally a nurse assigned to my patient would prove not to be a good match. One of the labor and delivery nurses in this story created tension for the whole family. When Lennie got an epidural, the nurse became less supportive and more patronizing. Ben tried to challenge her, the nurse was stubborn, and Lennie was busy having her baby.

We are only human, and nurses sometimes forget that experienced mothers know their bodies and should be trusted. Women in labor should be listened to carefully and believed.

If Lennie's training as an actor was part of her strength, helping her to focus and relax during labor, it also contributed to her disappointment. The birth scene wasn't played the way she wanted, and it was her only take. No do-overs. But Lennie learned to love the imperfection in her birth story. It is a good story.

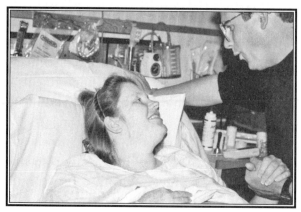

Lennie and Ben

LENNIE: When I was forty-one, we got pregnant again. We didn't plan it, but we weren't taking precautions either. We hemmed and hawed because our wealth has been a spiritual, social wealth, not financial. At that time it was all about caring about each other and being a family and being close. We had an amniocentesis because I was older and when we found out it was a boy, we were very, very happy. Both Ben and I had always wanted a boy.

The day of my baby shower was November 7th, and I was thirty-eight weeks pregnant. I went home and the reality hit that this baby was really going to be here soon. My blood pressure shot up and I started feeling ill the next morning. I had been watching what I ate and watching my blood pressure, but this was out of sight. I was put to bed, where I had to lie on my left side and keep my pressure down while I cooked this baby a while longer. I called on lots of friends to help with the girls, and I stayed on my side. I was very tired too, most of the time.

I think my blood pressure problem started when I realized that I was going to have a little boy. I hadn't dealt with that at all—my issues with men and boys and maleness. I just started freaking out. "Am I going to do it well? I want to do the best by him and give him what he needs to be a great man. Do I like men? Do I like boys? Where am I at with this issue? And God, I better start liking them because I'm going to have one." I spent a lot of the time on my side dealing with these issues and coming to peace with them.

We were starting to talk about inducing me close to my due date because of the blood pressure, and I knew things were already starting to happen. We tried to induce one day. My doctor put some gel in next to my cervix, and it didn't work, so she sent me home to wait a little longer. Ben wasn't as disappointed as I was because he wanted this baby to be born on the 22nd. He's an astrologer, and that was the date that made the most sense for our family.

Meanwhile, I was working with a hypnotherapist about the male issues. I hadn't been concerned with the other two births, but for this one I needed to have complete trust in myself to maneuver my way through to have a healthy baby. I didn't really have a mantra, or a specific thing to focus on. I just had to trust that I would know at every turn which decision to make in order to have a healthy baby. I didn't want to make an issue about having him naturally. I wanted to be open to all possibilities in every possible way to get the best result for me and the baby. Hypnosis helped me learn to make the right decisions from my gut, more than from my mind.

On the 22nd we started to induce again, and my blood pressure shot up. The baby's heart started doing some weird things. Stacey walked in the room saying, "Lennie, I'm going to say the 'C' word right now, right off the bat. It's in the realm of possibilities." I took a deep breath. There was something about having him pass through the birth canal that was a real important thing for the baby and me. I really wanted that for each of us.

I went back to the hypnosis stuff and said, "I'm going to let that in. I'm going to let that in. That's a possibility. It's not optimal for me or the baby, but I am going to have all the information I need to have." The nurse I had right then was wonderful, and she asked if I knew about epidurals. We had a wonderful conversation about what epidurals did.

When the situation is unstable (like with Lennie's blood pressure) and the baby is stressed, it is not a bad thing to mention the possibility of a Cesarean section. It can also be motivational, and I have seen many women work very hard to avoid surgery when faced with that possibility.

I got up and walked around, working my butt off. The contractions were getting more intense, and I wasn't dilating. My blood pressure started going up again, his heart did weird things again, and I decided the epidural was a good thing to try. One of the side effects of an epidural is low blood pressure. I figured I could use that.

The same anesthesiologist who gave me anesthesia during my knee operation came in and gave me the epidural. I felt completely empowered when I got that epidural and it felt really good. My communication with Stacey was really good. We could communicate on an intuitive level and that was important to me.

I had two nurses. One nurse was a very, very good one who would get quiet every time the other one would walk in. The other one treated me as if I'd given up my power with the epidural. She quit talking to me, she quit listening to me, and she dismissed me. It was as if she felt because I was drugged that she had to make the decisions. She was being patronizing, like she had her own agenda. That was a problem because Ben was not having a good time with her at all. There was this triad of Ben, this nurse, and me. I did not want to involve myself in the struggle, but I was watching her and Ben work it out and dealing with myself too.

Even though I had the epidural, I could still feel the contractions. I rested for about thirty minutes, but I felt the pain. They were not nearly as intense, but they were there. Then it became a big issue when I said, "Call my doctor *now.*" I wanted Stacey there right away. The nurse said, "Oh you still have to push." And I said, "No, you don't understand. I don't push. The baby is going to be here. *Call my doctor now.*" Thirty minutes went by and she came back in the room and I said, "Did you call my doctor?" She said, "No, I haven't called her yet but I'll call her in a few minutes." She made another excuse and again I looked at her and I said, "Call her now." I was pissed at that point, and she made a face at me and walked out of the room again.

Ben said, "Do you want me to do something?" And I said, "Let me see if she comes back in and says she called her." And she walked back in the room and said, "I called." I said, "The baby is coming now. The baby is going to be here now. It's now." And so she checked me and looked and said, "Yes, here it is! Don't push, don't push. Breathe!" And then she said to the other nurse, "Get the stuff." The other nurse said to her, "Are you going to call the doctor on call downstairs?" And she said, "No, I'm going to do this one myself. All she has to do is blow it out." The baby was coming so fast I had to kind of hold it back by blowing my breath some.

I am still pissed to this day about being disregarded. It was enough for me to manage myself and the baby. I didn't have any energy to fight with her. I didn't have the energy or presence of mind to say, "No, you get a doctor." I was really praying that my own doctor would come in the door

Always ask your doctor for her direct phone number. If necessary, you should be able to contact her without going through the nurses, especially if you are having difficulties like Ben and Lennie were experiencing.

any second. Which she did, about thirty seconds after the baby was born. It was a heartbreaker. I wanted her to be there and I wanted to look into her face. I didn't want a stranger who was power-tripping. I didn't want that energy there. And at the same time I didn't fight it because I wanted to be as present as I could possibly be. So I was trying to permit anything I had to deal with.

Despite all that, it was a beautiful birth: simple and quiet. I could feel my legs, I could feel everything. I felt him come out and he just slid out. I felt him, held him on my stomach, and rubbed him. It was really, really beautiful. I was encased in a bubble and that nurse couldn't get inside that bubble, but I wanted the bubble to be just more than me and Eyan. I wanted it to be the whole room. And it wasn't the whole room. I wish I had told someone that I needed a different nurse.

What's the lesson here? I think it has to do with surrendering and knowing that it was bigger than everybody. It was bigger than her. And it was knowing when to fight and when not to fight. I really did make the best decision at every turn for myself and the baby, and everything came out fine. Even though it wasn't totally perfect, there is something perfect about being just a little bit askew because that's real. And the acceptance of that thing that's a little askew felt good.

Eyan weighed six pounds, eleven ounces. He has been peaceful and joyful since he was born.

If a nurse is difficult to work with, remember that your birth is bigger than any unhelpful individual. Pay attention to your own process and don't let any one person get in the way of a satisfying birth. If it is intolerable, respectfully ask for a different nurse. (Remember: You do not lose your voice just because you are in a hospital.)

We aren't having any more kids because I'm too freakin' old! Ben finally had himself cut. We've talked about it, and we know if we had started when we were about ten years younger, we could have had eight or ten kids. We make beautiful, beautiful healthy gorgeous babies together. But we wanted to handle other projects, and we had other creative "births" to give.

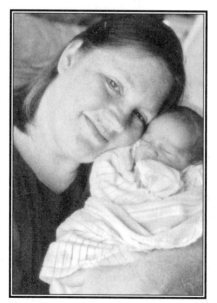

Lennie and Eyan

JESSE

BOBBI AND JESSE

Al and Bobbi are potters who raised three girls amidst the dust, glaze, and heat of a potter's studio. When their youngest daughter was fourteen, they had an unexpected pregnancy that turned into a lesson they are still learning to appreciate. This particular story does not have the happy ending we all expect and wish for. Not everyone gets to go home with a cuddly healthy baby, but every expectant mother does get to experience a birth.

Bobbi went into labor in her twenty-third week. This birth was managed with the midwifery model in a hospital. We could have been extremely invasive, using medications to stop labor and help the baby's lungs mature quickly. We could have transferred Bobbi to an intensive obstetric facility, but she did not want that kind of birth. She wanted no aggressive intervention, so we simply stayed with her and supported her and her family with compassion.

But this is not a story of The Worst. While it is true that Jesse was born too early to survive, Bobbi's pregnancy and birth was complete and full. She misses her son every day, but would not have missed having him in her life for all the world. This is a story of enduring love and incredible bravery. It is a story for women who want to know what it means to be strong, to be courageous, and to love with all their hearts, no matter what the cost may be.

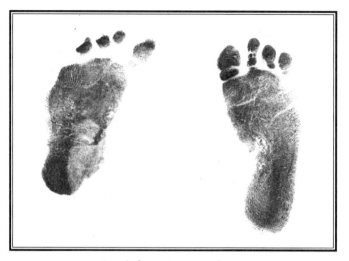

Jesse's footprints, actual size

BOBBI: This is the story of Jesse.

We chose the name Jesse because we thought it was a wonderful name and the energy would rub off on him. It was a biblical name and that meant a lot to Al. Old Testament. Maybe we knew early on that this was a very special energy, a very special soul, because it is a root name—the name Jesus came from—a very early Hebrew stock line. I know we hadn't thought it out—it was just the name it had to be, whether it was a boy or girl.

Getting pregnant was a surprise. My plate was really full at the time. I was working full time as a painting contractor, and Al was getting to the point where he needed more medical attention. He has a hip replacement from an old accident and it keeps him in pain most of the time. I was trying to balance all that, along with taking care of my teenage kids.

I had an IUD in place. Or not. It was a lost IUD. Five years before, I had been checked at a clinic and told that the IUD was not there and not to worry about it. No one did a sonogram, and I assumed they knew what they were talking about. I was also experiencing perimenopause symptoms. I was forty, my periods were lighter, and I was having temperature changes. When I stopped having periods, I went to see Stacey, took a pregnancy test, and was shocked. I had already given myself a home test and it came up positive, but I had talked myself into believing it wasn't real.

It had been fourteen years since I had been pregnant, and here I was two months along already. Al was forty-seven when we got pregnant. There was a question about whether I should have a D&C (dilation and curettage) because of the IUD, and just let the pregnancy go. Al was realistic about it and didn't say a whole lot. Although we both knew how we felt, he respected that this would be a woman's decision. So, he let me make the choice to keep the pregnancy. We were serious but also kind of excited.

We didn't do an amniocentesis, even though I was older, because I couldn't make that decision to have an abortion if there was anything wrong with the baby. When we did a sonogram for this pregnancy, we saw the IUD in there. I thought if I got past the second trimester I might be okay. It's a numbers game and we knew that. Besides the fact that the IUD made it a risky situation to begin with, my job didn't help, being so physically demanding. So I just had to accept that it'd either work or not.

I had a different feeling, a much darker feeling, with this pregnancy. I tend to try to cancel that out because you wonder which comes first, the dark feeling or the event, and you put that aside because you don't want to give yourself negative energy.

I had an excellent pregnancy. I felt the baby early on; we had communication, more of a spiritual space. It was really neat because we'd talk to each other and do things. I really didn't do that with the other kids. Each time, I loved being pregnant, but this one was sort of special. And you wonder if it's just because you knew this is the absolute last time you're ever going to be pregnant in your life, so you pay more attention. It was a good thing. Al's experience was the same, focused on being pregnant. And the baby was really focused on us.

I felt great and didn't get sick. I didn't have any of that kind of response to it, but I could tell the difference in my age. I didn't have as much energy. I felt tired, and that was harder.

We thought we had pretty much passed the point of concern until the twenty-third week. I knew when I was at work that we had hit the wall. I felt my entire body shift. I was carrying a large five-gallon paint can up to the second story and I started leaking amniotic fluid. Something just gave, and I thought, "This is stupid." But you know, it was one of those weird situations in your life when you don't have the luxury to stop. That just wasn't one of the options.

We called Stacey and went into the hospital. She checked me and said it was room-and-board time and I would be in for the duration, however long that was. We were trying to stop the leak, and I was starting to get contractions.

I had started to go into labor and was trying to put it aside, trying to slow it down and make an honest assault on changing the way things were going with my body. I knew the inevitable was happening but I owed myself the effort. We were within four days of having him be acceptable as a preemie, but I'm not sure if I would have intervened or made any changes. I think that's a terrible thing to do to a child, to start him off so hard.

It was just insane. All these people were there that night. I did not want to be cordial, and these people were there because they cared. So what do you do? I remember thinking, "I just wish they'd go away because I'm terrible company. There's business at hand and it's not working." I was trying to stay real calm because my kids were there, and I was trying not to let them see me sweat. I was trying to stay organized and look like I had a sense of control, which I didn't.

It was very hard. I don't really have icky labor. It is usually very short and productive. But this was like having nagging period cramps that wouldn't go away and knowing what it was: the Monster. It was a door, and I was saying, "No! No!"

I sent Al home. He understood that I needed to be by myself and he respected that. There was nothing he could do and it would be very distracting to have him there in that situation.

My Dad called after everyone left. It was a long-distance call and he talked and talked and talked to me. The whole time I was trying to sound like I was focusing on what he was saying, but I was thinking, "There is definitely something taking over my ability to concentrate. My body needs me to think." And it was probably the longest telephone call in the world. I have no idea how long it was, but I was afraid if I said there was something wrong, I would offend him or he would get very worried. I was trying to be very casual in talking to him and breathing at the same time and thinking, "Okay, I've lost the battle."

You wonder after the fact if giving yourself permission to lose the battle, you lose it, or if you lose it anyway and just mentally accept it.

Anyway, later that evening, it went from just having persistent cramping to definite contractions, and then to realizing that there was no way I could hold back.

I told the nurse. All the signs were obvious that the baby was coming: My water was there, and the contractions came often. I knew whatever the outcome, Al wanted to be there, but how to get hold of him was another situation. He was at the neighbor's house and our phone was busy, so we couldn't get through.

DR. KERR: This was the only time that I have ever called the operator and asked her to cut into another call. We had to get hold of Al and get him to the hospital in time for this birth. The operator cut in, I talked to Al, and he and their daughter were able to be there within fifteen minutes.

BOBBI: I guess basically I'm a control freak, and it stuck in my mind about how tenuous our hold is on our control, and how hard it is to acknowledge the fact that you've gone over the line. So, no matter how much you don't want the outcome to happen, at a certain point you just go out gracefully. Or big-time ungracefully.

It was very easy to deliver him. He was very tiny, just a plop out of me. It was nothing. It was really interesting because we had been so connected all along. Even if his life signs were failing, I could tell his spirit was so strong and so much bigger than he was. He was just this little toy thing. Tiny. We wrapped him up and we held him. He held on to my finger which was painful at the time, but in the long run, it was really healing.

I've always had a special connection with my children, but especially with him because I had to acknowledge and face what it was. It definitely is a spiritual thread that runs back and forth between the parent and the child. He had such an enormous energy field around him that was pure light. Here he was, a little one pound, three ounce child reaching out and grabbing hold of my finger. I was bathed in energy from him as his body slowed down and finally stopped functioning. I could feel his energy stretching out almost like it was thinning. It was moving away, and yet it was still connected to my hand. It was really neat, wonderful, and warm.

I can still cry.

At a certain point, I had to make a choice whether I was going to go with him or stay. It only lasted a few minutes, maybe seconds, but it seemed like forever. And I remember thinking to myself that it was my role to stay. I had to stay because I had stuff to do. I had a lot of other people that I was connected to, and that was a really sad part, the choice. And I remember taking his fingers off of my finger, opening up his little hand. I was disconnecting myself from that, the physical connection with him. It was a very hard tactile disengagement and it leaves a hole. I'm sure many other people have experienced this when people they are close to leave this realm. But it's still a very personal dark hole. Al experienced this also. At the time it was just my own little dark hole, but we were all experiencing it.

There wasn't a lot of time to go searching for the little spirit that was out there because I had a daughter and husband who were there participating in this experience with me, who were needy, and I felt myself shifting to gather ourselves up. The mom thing.

I had to stay the night to make sure I was not going to bleed, and they were kind enough to put me in a room away from the other mothers and newborns. I was trying to go to sleep and be all by myself. Such a change. On one hand it was good, I'm sure, and on the other hand I was disoriented and it was way too much. I should have been home. The next morning, I had my bags packed and was on the edge of the bed waiting for Al to come and get me.

It was really hard because we truly had anticipated and wanted this child. We'd made a conscientious, thought-out choice about this. And then there was no choice. So it was difficult to rationalize why we could lose the baby. It took me a number of years to get to the point where I could talk about it and look for the good things, to try and find where the blessings are. It didn't look like much of a blessing to me at the beginning.

Some people like to share the thought of a spiritual soul presence, and some people are not comfortable with that. I was a little intimidated by it and hadn't said anything about it. I had a friend who called from out of state the day after Jesse died. She said, "I prayed all night that you would stay." I said, "What are you talking about?" And she said, "I felt that you were leaving with the baby." And she didn't even know that I was miscarrying.

I am no great philosopher or theologian, but there is something out there—something a heck of a lot bigger than we are. I'm not a fantasy person, not on that level. One of the reasons I have a hard time imagining Jesse now is because I so totally do not feel comfortable around angels and that kind of stuff. I can't think of a human manifestation of a spirit. But I am very humbled to have shared those moments and the time I was pregnant with that soul. It was quite an amazing gift to have shared that time. I have felt spirits leave before, but I have never seen that light before. I think I saw it because his was so pure and I was just experiencing, not judging.

To this day I have to catch myself when I feel as though I could have done something different. *If* I had been more together, I would have found my instincts and I would have had a second opinion on the IUD. *If* I had quit working and kept my feet up in the air for nine months, I wouldn't have lost him. *If* I hadn't been so pigheaded and had somebody else carry those buckets of paint, he would still be here. But my heart just gets to a certain point, and I know I did the best I could do at the time. Maybe I'm just one of those people who have to run their head into a wall. I don't think a lot about myself physically and I don't give myself limitations. This is definitely the first time in my life that it ever backfired on me. And I still do that. I can't say that I'm reformed, but I have a sad memory to go with it now. I don't know how I could really have changed that because that was who I was, and that was what I did. I would encourage people, if they're able, to know themselves a little better than I did.

I think there is a gift in all of this. There is a balance. Really rotten things happen, but I don't think they come without gifts. They are not always the gifts we are looking for. Even though I don't see him as an entity, there is probably not a day that goes by that he doesn't pop up in my mind, and it's not because I'm mourning or anything. I remember what I felt during that time and something that he triggered in me. He left us with a much deeper sense of our own potential, our spiritual value, and our soul value. It gives me hope that this is something to look forward to in this life and that I will see my own potential.

It's an incredible example of how pure we are when we are first born. We have this huge, pure spirit poured into this tiny little tin can. The vessel Jesse was in wasn't big enough for the spirit. But he stuck around long enough to say, "Howdy," and that was good.

I have not felt that same energy again. I think you are always out there with your radar looking for that spirit. I know there was a point to his life. It was a strong point. He did some pretty earth-shaking things in the very short time he was here. His life definitely had more impact on me than anyone's life has ever had and made me think and rethink, wrestling with a lot of issues that I would have put on the back burner.

If Jesse were here in this room with us today, what would you say to him?

I'd ask him to give me his hand back. He doesn't have to say anything, just hold my hand.

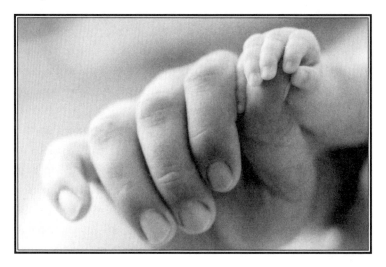

Angels on My Shoulder

Deborah and Gavin

Deborah and Mike had their second baby about three and a half years after their first son, Dylan, was born. Deborah's delivery with Dylan had been difficult. He was a very large baby, and his shoulders got stuck on the way out (shoulder dystocia). It took all my strength and skill to manipulate that baby out of his mother, head out, body still inside, face turning purple as the seconds ticked away while I twisted first one way, then the other, pulling steadily. It is the moment most of us who catch babies dread: a significant shoulder dystocia. I did get him out, without complications. And actually, Dylan did well once he was born, but my arms and hands were trembling too much to hold the glass of celebratory champagne, much less sign the birth certificate right after his delivery.

Deborah was pregnant again, and an early blood-sugar lab test had diagnosed gestational diabetes. Within weeks we realized that diet alone was not going to control Deborah's blood sugars, so we had to teach her to inject herself with daily insulin. The complicated and challenging task of monitoring her diet, insulin, and blood sugars consumed most of Deborah's time and energy for the second half of the pregnancy. She is a generous Italian woman who loves to eat, so maintaining her regimen was no small challenge.

Deborah was not worried about this birth. Her ability to manage her diet and blood sugar gave her confidence, and she was eagerly looking forward to meeting her son. I, however, was concerned. Her dependence on insulin made her high risk, and she had a history of shoulder dystocia. I wanted everything to go well, but I knew we would require some medical help in Deborah's childbirth to manage her diabetes and deliver a potentially big baby.

At each visit, Deborah, Mike, and I would talk about her diabetes control, how she was feeling, and possible birth plans. I told them what to expect at the hospital this time so they would not be surprised by the extra medical attention. Certainly she would need an IV during labor to help manage her blood sugar, and induction was a possibility we discussed as she neared her due date. We laughed about my refusal to induce this baby before the year end, saying that the tax break was not worth the medical intervention. Throughout our discussions, Deborah had the final say in all decisions. Our birth choices were made carefully, always looking for the balance between trusting Mother Nature and providing necessary intervention.

Here is Deborah's story. My own story follows—of the same birth, but told from my point of view. Same ending, though: Gavin Albert Reid—born January 13, 2004 and weighing seven pounds, thirteen ounces.

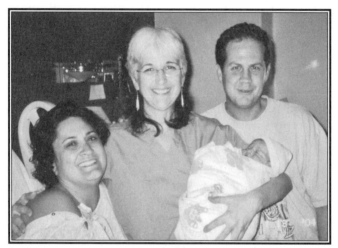

Deborah, Dr. Kerr, Gavin, and Mike

DEBORAH: I was due on January 18th and entered the hospital on January 11th. We wanted to make sure it wasn't as big of a baby as my first child. We had done several tests and they were measuring anywhere between six and nine pounds. Dylan weighed nine pounds, six ounces, and that was just *too* big. So we all agreed that inducing labor would be a good idea.

I was nervous and a little scared, not because of birth but because of the induction process and not knowing what to expect. So we started with pills on my cervix; first we did two of those. I felt nothing. That night we let the pills take their course, but they weren't doing much. My cervix was high and kind of mushy but not ready, not open. At six in the morning, we decided to forget the pills and go with the Pitocin. We started the IV then, but the Pitocin did not do anything. I slept until about noon, which the nurses thought was very unusual. So we backed off the Pitocin and went back to the pills on the cervix.

We did two more pill insertions, waiting four hours in between. About four in the afternoon, almost immediately after we did that second and final pill, my water broke. I was sort of expecting things to come on really strong like they did before when my water broke. With Dylan, the contractions were really heavy and I could feel myself moving into labor more, but this time I didn't. It was different. I did some walking and felt some contractions, but they weren't incapacitating. They weren't strong enough to bring the cervix down enough. So we started Pitocin around six that night again. Instead of going backwards it was time to forge ahead. We were not leaving without a baby!

Inducing childbirth is not like jump starting a car. Sometimes the body is simply not ready and no matter how much Pitocin we give, contractions don't happen. If the membranes are ruptured and Pitocin does not bring on contractions, the baby must be born by Cesarean section. On the other hand, if the waters are intact, you can always go home, wait a few days, and try again. It usually works the second time around, and then you have avoided major surgery.

When we started doing the Pitocin again, things started really heating up. I had some pretty serious pains, greater than I had ever experienced with Dylan, who was born without any pain medication. I felt like I had handled this portion of it before, so why wasn't I able to handle it now? I was having a hard time seeing the light at the end of the tunnel and was not able to work through the contractions like I wanted to. That's why I almost immediately started asking for pain medication.

I got the go ahead for an injection of Nubain. It helped, but not enough. It took the edge off a little bit, but the contractions were coming on stronger then, and faster, so fast that I couldn't regain focus in between and that's when I started asking for more medicine.

It is not always helpful to know how dilated your cervix is, especially if it is not what you hoped for or what you expect. Sometimes it is best not to know, especially since we never know how fast the cervix is going to open up.

I was told that I was three to four centimeters dilated, so I got discouraged in my quest to do this without drugs and decided that I wanted more of what she had just given me, and I wanted to call the anesthesiologist for the epidural. I waited for a while and got another injection, which took the edge off. Barely. Then we moved from the prelabor room to the actual delivery room, and by the time I got from one to the other, just across the hall, the anesthesiologist was there.

Getting the epidural was kind of creepy. I remember having to sit up very still and concentrate on not feeling the pain. I could feel him putting the needle in, a little pressure there, and I could feel him with the tubing—not something I wanted to feel but something I chose to feel at the time. It was a little bit of pressure and then some funny internal feelings, the tubing that was going in. He had a little trouble finding the spot and took a little longer getting it in place, and I could feel that. Then once it took over that was pretty much the end of feeling any pain down there, from my hips down. But I could still feel the pressure that was building as Gavin moved into place. I still felt the need to push.

During the epidural, I had uncontrolled shaking. I could talk but I wasn't really interested in conversation. I was really cold. They wanted to warm me up with all these towels. I just had this uncontrollable need to shake. That kind of put me in a funny place but I was able to work through that.

Once I got the epidural I lay back down, and *then* she checked me. I was at nine centimeters and feeling the urge to push a little bit. That was about an hour and a half between three to four centimeters and eight to nine. I look back now and know that was why it hurt so badly. I could've handled a steady, gradual dilation. I don't think they realized how fast it was going. It was in part because I was lying down and the contractions were coming on so hard that I didn't think I could get up and walk around. But the minute I got up to make the trek across the hall it really brought him down and put him into the birth canal even heavier. I had to move.

Sitting up for the epidural allowed the baby's head to apply itself to the cervix. This was very helpful and Deborah's shaking was indicating a fast and effective labor.

The epidural gave me a little bit of a reprieve, where I could think not just about pain but about what I needed to do to have the baby. The pain before the epidural was a full ten on a scale of one to ten, like no other pain I had felt before. I was surprised at that. I had been through labor and thought I knew what it was like, but the pain was not anything close to what I knew. And it was definitely *pain* pain. It wasn't nerves; I don't think I was scared or anything like that. It was just hard and fast pain. I felt it with each contraction in and around the lower half of my abdomen.

After the epidural, there wasn't much pain. There was pressure, because I felt like I needed to push. And I could feel things were progressing. I could feel I had a better handle on what my body was doing. I

Remember, just as every child is unique, so is every labor and delivery.

could visualize the opening and that he was moving down.

I could control the urge to push. My focus moved to, "Why is my body reacting this way to the medication? Why am I uncontrollably shaking?" I was shaking until I was actually able to push. Then I would take a minute, regain focus, and then my whole body would shake again. The anesthesiologist hung around a little while, and I think that might have set my nerves off because I was thinking, "What does he want with me?" He was done and as I recall we had done an internal fetal monitor. I was really not interested in doing one of those at the time but was urged by people there to do it because we were having trouble keeping an eye on Gavin's status. And my blood pressure was doing funny things so

The anesthesiologist usually stays around for a while after placing an epidural, partly to make sure it was effective and partly to watch for side effects. Deborah's shakes probably made him a bit uneasy, because he didn't realize it was all due to a fast labor.

I think that was why the anesthesiologist hung out. But that is all hearsay because I just don't recall!

Once the nurse checked me after the epidural, it was clear to her that things were going to go along pretty quickly and that is when she called Dr. Kerr.

There were eight people there. Most had been there all day, off and on—my mother, my sister, my fourteen-year-old niece, my husband, and three friends. But for the most part, it was my sister and husband during the really heavy pain of it all. My sister was the one who helped me through it, just like when I had Dylan. She helped me focus and kept me from going over the edge. She did a pretty good job of it.

When Dr. Kerr showed up, I felt like I was ready to get on with this. I was still shaking—intermittent bouts of uncontrollable shaking. Pushing was a breeze. I thank Dylan for that, for forging the way. It was two pushes and Gavin was out, all seven pounds, thirteen ounces of him. I was surprised. I was overjoyed it was going so fast. I could feel it. I knew it was going to be fast even before Dr. Kerr came because I could feel him moving into position. The epidural was a good feeling that way. It was definitely a different feeling than with Dylan, when I pushed and pushed and couldn't really feel it.

It was weird that I had the urge to push this time. I didn't last time. But I could handle the contractions last time and couldn't handle them this time. It was just all very different. I have to think that the intensity was due to the Pitocin induction because it was the exact opposite of what I experienced during a normal, uninduced labor. My water broke at four in the afternoon, hard contractions started at seven or eight in the evening, and he was born at twelve thirty in the morning on the 13th. Four hours to do it all. Overload.

I was not worried about the shoulders. We were a week early, and I felt like I had much better control of the entire scenario since I got diagnosed with diabetes. I knew there had to be a pot of gold at the end of that rainbow!

I felt smaller throughout the pregnancy. I was losing weight instead of gaining weight, and that was a good indicator for me that things were going to be different this time.

Was it fun? It wasn't the most fun thing I've ever done in my life, but I got to take the prize home. It wasn't *not* fun. It just was.

Regrets? I have none. Well, I wish I'd have moved to the delivery room and sat up longer and maybe not have needed the epidural. I got so discouraged. I wished she hadn't said the number three when she checked my cervix that first time. It may have been just psychological, but knowing the number really discouraged me. Had I gotten up and moved across the hall even, and sat up and had to focus. . . But it was the choice I made at the time I was told three centimeters, and maybe it was a good choice because it gave me a few minutes of relaxation before the big push. And that was how it had to be.

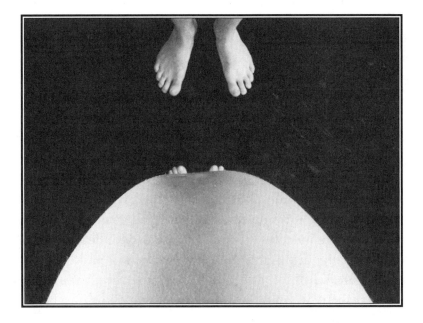

My advice to others is to embrace it, and that is all you can do. You can't control it, and as much as you want to, you have no choice and you have to let go. Control the things you can control and don't worry about the things you can't, which is what I try to remember in my entire life! It's a life lesson.

※

DR. KERR: The first rule of delivering babies is Hold No Fear. Fear causes complications. I knew better, but couldn't help myself. I was worried. This was scary stuff, and I was feeling the pressure.

I couldn't shake the memory of Dylan's difficult birth, and in the recesses of my mind, tucked away for no one else to see, was the fear that this time I wouldn't be able to get Debbie's baby out safely. Each time that niggling fear crept in, I would shove it back and remind myself that I had no room for fear. This was a new pregnancy, no reason to worry about the same thing happening. It could be easier this time.

Halfway through her pregnancy, we had to start Deb on insulin shots for gestational diabetes. "Great," I said to myself, "Insulin-dependent gestational diabetic with history of shoulder dystocia on previous pregnancy." This did not look good. Per the protocol, I had to call a specialist for back up.

Dr. F wasn't worried when I called. This was the kind of pregnancy he handled all the time. Of course, he hadn't been there when Dylan was born. On the other hand, insulin generally keeps the baby smaller and that would likely make the delivery easier. Deb was using more insulin every week and watching her diet like a hawk.

At each visit with Mike and Debbie, I reassured them about the birth, and as we got closer to the due date we discussed their options. I had frequent telephone consultations with Dr. F, and when Deb was thirty-seven weeks pregnant, I ordered an amniocentesis. Testing the amniotic fluid would enable me to see if the baby's lungs were developed enough to induce labor. Inducing labor goes against my usual philosophy of "Let Mother Nature call the shots." But because the mom was an insulin-dependent diabetic whose belly was already large enough to be at term, I stepped in to help Mother Nature along.

The radiologist was unable to get the amniotic fluid. The placenta was in the way, and the baby wouldn't allow any space to safely insert the needle. So we agreed to wait a while longer before inducing.

We waited. I put my fear out of my mind. Finally, a week before her calendar due date, we agreed to induce labor.

We had to "ripen" the cervix with medication before we could start any Pitocin, and there was always the possibility that the ripening process would start effective labor all by itself. However, that was not to be. It took almost two days of ripening and IV Pitocin to start real labor, but Deb was not willing to back off; she was not going to let this baby get any bigger. Patience and persistence are virtues during this part of the process.

Finally, the induction worked. I knew I could be called in from home at any time to catch this baby. The heart rate was fine; the nurses told me that Deb was doing well and had requested an epidural. We had all agreed that if we needed to use Pitocin, she would be given any other medications she needed to handle the pain of induced labor. There would be no question about an epidural. She would get one whenever she asked for it.

I knew I needed to get some sleep before I delivered this child, but I was having trouble drifting off. Fear was my companion that night. It was my responsibility to banish it completely—it had no business visiting the birth of this baby. But how could I rid myself of the fear?

As I tossed and turned, I focused my thoughts on my years of delivering babies. I remembered the sure knowledge that there were angels attending each birth, surrounding the event with safety and a spiritual presence. I also remembered the moment I first felt I was flying solo without the full support of guardian angels. It was a birth shortly after that fateful September 11th in 2001.

That night I was walking the hallways of the hospital while the mother labored and was trying to sort out my feelings. Why was I feeling uneasy? Why was I less certain of a good birth this time around? It felt like it was up to me to make the birth safe, that the angels were busy elsewhere. The births after that day had been a little bit difficult for me, and I wondered if my guardian angels would ever make themselves felt again.

Tonight I needed my angels back. Heck, I didn't want to do this birth without the full team that had accompanied me all those years! I knew I could do it without them, but I missed them, now more than ever. They could help banish my fear. So as I lay in bed that night, I visualized huge white angel wings, larger than me, at least seven feet long, that opened like a nest to surround me. The wings cradled me in their softness and I felt supported and secure. Warmth and safety enveloped me. I slept.

The phone rang, jerking me awake. Just an hour after I'd ordered the epidural, Deb was fully dilated and ready to push. I leaped out of bed, stumbled to the bathroom, and brushed my teeth. As I drove to the hospital, the midnight streets deserted and the town sound asleep, I felt again the anxiety and fear of what I would have to do to get us all through this safely. I grabbed for those wings and draped them over my shoulders like a cape, using my visualization skills to drive away the images of possible complications awaiting me.

The room was full of people. I am not exaggerating—there were at least eight people in the room when I arrived. It felt like a party, so I focused on Deborah's face. "Are you ready?" I asked.

"I guess so," she said with a big smile.

"I will be right back after I change for this occasion!" I went to change into scrubs and when I returned a few minutes later, there were fewer people in the room and the energy was more focused. It was time to push this baby out. I put on my gloves and sat down to work, checking the position of the baby's head and reviewing the heart rate, a good indicator of baby distress.

Smiling reassuringly at Deborah, I took a deep breath, drew my angel's wings closely around my shoulders, and extended those wings in my mind's eye to encompass both her and Mike. I asked her to start pushing. Black hair was visible. I called Mike to come see the first view of his baby's head. He watched as the head moved easily down the birth canal, and two pushes later the head was out. No waiting this time. Another push, and all of Gavin Reid fell into my hands as smooth as silk.

With sure hands I placed him on Deborah's belly where he gave us those wonderful lusty cries we love to hear. It was the most beautiful birth I could have hoped for, surrounded by friends and family, and attended by my guardian angels once again. I had wrestled with fear and won. What a precious prize for winning!

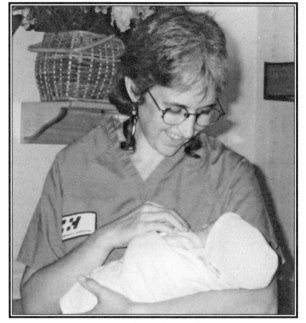

Dr. Kerr with a beloved prize

JUST DO IT

LUCY AND CHRISTOPHER AND KATELYN

Lucy was thirty-seven and Ken was thirty-eight when Lucy gave birth to Christopher and Katelyn. Lucy is a level-headed woman full of common sense, born and raised in Canada. She was a perfect candidate for a midwifery model birth, but because she was carrying twins, I consulted with an obstetric specialist during the pregnancy and labor. The medical model played a role almost from the beginning. Lucy is pragmatic, willing to do whatever it takes to get the job done.

Although the situation required extensive medical intervention, Lucy did not complain. It was our constant communication that made this birth integrative. Frequent visits, open discussions about the pregnancy and labor, and the personal attention of her doctors kept Lucy informed and involved.

An integrative physician also has the humility to learn valuable lessons from each birth. Lucy's birth reminded me to honor a mother's need to see her babies as soon as they are born. When births are primarily techno-medical, we may too easily overlook a mother's fears—fears that are only relieved when a new mother sees her baby and knows all is well. The more technology is involved in birth, the more a physician must consciously respect the family's emotional needs.

Prenatal care when a woman is carrying twins is quite different than for a single baby. We had to make sure that one of the twins wasn't stealing all the nutrients from the placenta and depriving the other of its chance to thrive. We did numerous sonograms as Lucy's due date came closer, measuring both babies to make sure they were growing equally and sharing their space. The last sonogram, done about three weeks before the delivery, indicated that the babies were within a few ounces of each other.

This story illustrates once again Mother Nature's sense of humor. Despite our best medical expertise, our estimate of the comparative size of these two babies was way off, much to everyone's surprise on the day of their birth. No, I take that back. The babies knew there was a big difference. It just took the rest of us a while to realize what was going on.

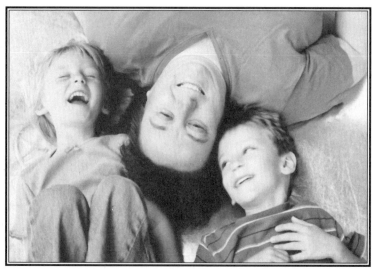

Katelyn, Lucy, and Christopher

LUCY: We had talked about getting pregnant for a couple of months. Andrew, Ken's son, was twelve, and we weren't sure we wanted to have a baby since he was going to be grown and gone pretty soon. I had been pregnant once before and had miscarried. We had been married for a year, and I thought, "If I don't do it now..." Mind you, my mother didn't start having babies until her mid-thirties and continued well into her mid-forties, so I wasn't concerned about age because I'm fit. It was more of an issue of Ken and I having time together.

I went off the pill and I was pregnant within two months. We thought it was going to take a while and had planned to move to a bigger house. We didn't want to get pregnant until maybe a year after we actually started trying, but it turned out okay.

I felt sick and my breasts hurt, so I came to Dr. Kerr's office for a pregnancy test. I was about four weeks along. I didn't feel sick for very long, but the first trimester was very strange. At first we thought maybe we had the wrong date because the morning sickness stopped so early and I gained ten pounds in the first month. I thought maybe I wasn't feeling well because I wasn't riding my bike. Normally I would ride about one hundred and fifty to two hundred miles a week.

We got a sonogram because we were unsure about the dates, and the last thing on my mind was that I was having twins. There are no twins in either family. Even when I got the sonogram, I thought it was a split screen and I was just seeing the same fetus twice. I really did!

"We have twins!"

"We what?"

Both Ken and I were sitting there. It was Ken's birthday, too. It sure took a bit of getting used to! I was in shock driving back to work and all that day. When I got home, we were both dazed.

Our alpha-fetoprotein (AFP) blood test came back abnormal, even for twins, and we had to go get an amniocentesis. That wasn't as bad as I thought it was going to be, because everybody says that it hurts so much and it really doesn't. I mean, it hurts like a bee sting. So it wasn't bad. They had a problem with one because the placenta was on top and they had to go through it to get to the sack. He tested Christopher, put dye in to avoid testing the same one twice, and came out. Then he tested Katelyn.

Getting an amniocentesis is a choice, not a requirement. It is a procedure that carries a small amount of risk to the pregnancy, so it must be well considered. But Lucy wanted to know and be prepared for any abnormalities, so she chose to accept the risk and get the test done.

I was terrified. I thought they would both have Downs syndrome, the double whammy. I was in tears every night. I could hold it together all day at work, but even that was hard because everyone knew I was waiting for news. The dialogue was, "Have you heard yet?" and, "No, I don't want to talk about it right now. Leave me alone." I would just lose it by the end of the day. It was ten days before we got the results. Ken called Dr. Kerr's office and said I was going crazy, so she called the lab directly to get the

One of the problems with amniocentesis is the anxiety of waiting for results. Make sure your provider will call you as soon as the results are available, and try to find out just when that might be. Don't be shy about asking for answers.

results. We found out the babies were both okay and what they were, boy and girl. The rest of the pregnancy was a breeze, emotionally.

That last month of pregnancy was very tiring because of the weight. I was huge, and it was uncomfortable to do anything. Ken cleaned the house and I'd come home and go to bed. I'd put my feet up, watch TV, and fall asleep.

I worked until three days before I went into labor. I'm an accountant, but I was up and about at work a fair amount, which was good. I was getting some exercise with walking, but I wasn't lifting. The kitchen was a fair distance from my office and I was drinking a lot of water. The people at work would leave the bathroom by my office open for me because when I had to go, I had to get in there and get in there fast.

I knew that with twins, I would likely deliver about three weeks early, so I quit work about three weeks before my due date. I had been home for three days when I woke up one morning and thought I would just stay in bed. I had done way too much the day before and thought I was just tired. I was going to get up and pack my bag for the hospital and get everything ready. That was my plan for that day, but it never got done.

When I woke up I had a cramp, like a menstrual cramp. Then a couple more. That's all it was. And I thought, "Something's adjusting." No big deal. When I got up I wasn't sure if my water had broken or if I had just lost control. I really didn't know. So I smelt it and there was no smell. And I thought, "Well, okay. Maybe the amount of water I've been drinking is just flying through my system." It leaked for a while, so I paged Ken, "I think I'm in labor. I'm not sure though. Nothing hurts. I just think my water broke." So he says, "Well, let me know. Get yourself down to the hospital."

I didn't call anyone else. I thought by the time I reached someone who could take me there, they'd be swarming all over me, and I hate that. Then when I got to the hospital, I got mad because I couldn't find a parking spot. I never thought about pulling up by the front door and having my vehicle moved later. They told me they would have done that but I didn't know.

There was a man there who had just pulled into a spot and I asked him, "Please, I'm in labor. Can I please have that spot because I've been driving around for a while!" and he just said, "No." And I just felt like ramming him with my Suburban. I thought, "You ruthless jerk!" So I went and parked down the street and walked to the hospital. And when I walked in, one of the admitting people noticed I was in labor and got me a wheelchair.

By that time I was having more cramps. I never thought they would be that mild. It was shocking because I really thought that they would be a lot stronger. They took me upstairs and did that paper test. "Yep, that was your water." And I started leaking again.

Then the contractions got bad, fast. The only thing I could think of was just trying to get through each one of those. I was trying to be natural and just get through them, but when they told me I was only two centimeters dilated, I got depressed. I got some medicine, and it worked for a little while. It calmed me down. I felt the contractions in the front and back. I don't know if that's possible or what, but it sure felt like it. I had either Ken or my sister-in-law pushing on my back as much as I could.

It seemed like I dealt with this forever. I have a high tolerance level for pain. And it hurt. They came so fast, one right after the other. It felt like they were continuous.

It's probably not the smartest plan to drive yourself to the hospital when you are in labor. Even though it may feel like early labor, you never know how it's going to go, and it is safer to have someone else drive.

Nitrazine paper will turn dark blue if it contacts amniotic fluid. We look into the vagina with a speculum and if fluid is pooling in there, we touch it with the paper and watch for the color change.

As we saw earlier, knowing how dilated your cervix is can be discouraging. Although we know the cervix can open up to ten centimeters in a very short amount of time, being told you are only two centimeters while you are having strong contractions is difficult. Because of this, some women would rather not know how dilated they are.

DR. KERR: When we checked her cervix after another hour or two, it was still only three centimeters dilated and the babies were still very high in her pelvis. The obstetrics specialist who was consulting had no idea why she wasn't dilating with all those contractions. It didn't make sense to me either. She was handling labor well and it all looked like it should be progressing.

So far we had managed to have a relatively noninterventional birth, other than the single dose of Nubain, but what we were doing wasn't working. After we discussed the situation with Lucy and Ken, we all agreed to give her an epidural and use Pitocin to stimulate labor that would hopefully bring the babies down and dilate the cervix.

LUCY: Getting the epidural was hard. I felt sorry for the doctor trying to get it in because the contractions were so bad and I was so tense. I couldn't relax, I was sweaty, and I had to arch my back and round it. I couldn't do that because my stomach was so large. I didn't realize that I'd have to do that. My stomach felt like it was twice the size of normal.

There's quite a misconception with epidurals that they are dangerous to get. I don't know if they are, but that's just what you hear. But when you experience that kind of pain, you don't even care. I wanted out of that situation. Maybe if I had made great progress and was closer to delivering, I would have tried to do without it. I do wish I would have had the opportunity to do it naturally, because I'm never going to have it again and it would have been nice to have one that way.

I felt like I was cut short because I went through all that work, I got to that point, and then there was nothing. I got my children, but it was very anticlimactic. But by that time I was feeling so sick that I had to do something.

I did sleep after I got the epidural, but Ken said I would whimper every time there was a contraction. I sort of knew what was going on around me but not totally.

DR. KERR: Two hours later, Lucy had a fever, she was shaking all over, and she really felt horrible. The twin on top, Christopher, had a dangerously rapid heart rate of 210 for about half an hour. After talking with Ken and Lucy, we decided do to a Cesarean section.

If labor is too painful, and you are unable to relax in between contractions, then you are less likely to be able to open up for the baby. Sometimes an epidural allows a woman to relax enough to let the contractions do an effective job of bringing the baby down and dilating the cervix.

I still did not understand why things were playing out this way, but often the answer becomes clear during the surgery. I could only hope it made sense once we had the babies out safe and sound.

LUCY: I tried to push a little, but I was having a hard time just getting some muscle control to do that. Dr. Kerr said I could try pushing for a little while to see if things changed, but if they didn't I'd still have to have a C-section. And I said, "No, let's go now." I had to move to the operating table, and I was feeling very nauseated. They just couldn't move me. They said, "Lift your butt and move yourself over," and there I was having contractions with sixty-five pounds sitting on my spine. Everything was confusing. There were a lot of people around and a

In spite of all our attempts to support a vaginal birth, the top twin was clearly in distress. Everyone agreed that delivering these babies with surgery was the safest and most compassionate plan.

lot of masks on. I really didn't know who was around me—I could see just eyes. I remember talking to the anesthesiologist about where I could still feel things. I'd been in labor for seventeen hours.

It didn't hurt having the babies delivered. It felt like a release of pressure when they came out. And it wasn't any more so when the second one came out. It didn't feel like I was hollow, just like the pressure was released. I saw the babies as they were being taken out of the operating room, but I don't know how long after they were delivered that was. It seemed like an awfully long time.

No one should take your baby away without you getting a chance to see it first, unless there is a need for immediate resuscitation. Even in a Cesarean section, the mother or the father should get to see the baby the minute it is born.

I was worried because the first thing I heard was, "Oh my gosh—she's so small!" I thought that there was something wrong with her. I just wanted to see if she was okay. I had heard all of these horror stories that they take the babies away and you don't get to see them if there is something wrong. So if you don't see them, then there is something wrong. And with everything I went through before, knowing that the tests weren't 100 percent, there is always that thing in the back of your mind that says that there still could be something wrong. I never thought about it until that moment.

In getting ready for this birth, my Mom was a big help to me. She set an example for me while I was growing up. She made me realize that you really can do anything you set your mind to. She also showed me that you just do what you have to do. Whatever life throws at you, you do it. I had training as an athlete too, and that helped me a lot, that discipline. It's hard to describe. You just have to do something and you don't think about it. You don't have to worry about it. You just do it.

DR. KERR: We needed to use some oxygen and warmth to support both of the twins after the stresses of an unproductive labor. Christopher weighed more than six pounds and Katelyn was barely four pounds, which was a whopping two pound difference! So much for the sonograms. After the birth, I saw that Christopher was quite big enough to come out, but Katelyn was blocking his exit. She, smaller and still not quite ready, was definitely uncooperative about moving down and out while he was aggressively pushing from above. We resolved the "disagreement" with our Cesarean section.

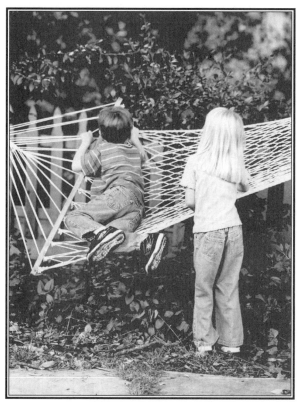

Christopher and Katelyn

CANCER CAN'T WAIT

CAROL AND LOGAN

Not at all interested in a homebirth? Neither was Carol. Some women make the choice to take full advantage of what modern medicine has to offer. During her first pregnancy, Carol passed her estimated due date without going into labor. When she was two weeks overdue, we agreed to induce her. She was huge, she was very ready to have her baby, and she was willing to accept the consequences of an induction.

Carol knew that she was committed to having her baby on that particular day. It didn't matter to her what it took, and she was not afraid of having a C-section. In fact, she was more afraid of going through labor than she was of surgery. She had no hesitation when I suggested we break her membranes to help induce her. Fourteen hours later, after we had tried cervical gel and Pitocin to no avail, Carol delivered by C-section.

Ashley was a huge baby, almost eleven pounds. No one questioned the need for a C-section when they saw this gorgeous baby girl, looking several weeks old the day after she was born.

Some women, once they have had a Cesarean, will decide to plan and schedule all their future births that way also. They have no desire to birth vaginally, and they like the control of an operative delivery. Carol had considered a vaginal birth after her first Cesarean, but it was not to be.

Her second pregnancy was complicated; she was told she had cervical cancer the same week she was told she was pregnant with a long awaited baby. The decisions she had to make were difficult, and at some point she gave up control to the doctors who were managing her cancer and her pregnancy. Her biggest choice came in the beginning when she decided to continue with her pregnancy in spite of the risks.

How does a physician like me fit into such a complex medical situation? As Carol's family physician, her pediatrician, and her advocate, I supported her decisions, answered her questions, and talked with her about her fears, which were many. Carol's fears shaped most of her experience. I trusted the specialist who was treating her cervical cancer and helping us manage the pregnancy. We worked together to provide the least invasive but safest experience we could for Carol.

Still, it was with mixed feelings that I managed Logan's birth. My goal as a physician was to make sure both mother and baby came through the pregnancy and birth in good health. My interest as an integrative physician was to encourage Carol to feel empowered through her birth experience. Her births gave her little opportunity to feel her strength, to enjoy the hormone-induced ecstasy of a natural labor, or to experience birth as an intense process that begins deep within a woman. Rather, her lessons were those of patience and trust in others.

Carol was blessed. Modern medicine provided her a safe birth and a healthy son and effectively treated her cancer. She was extremely brave and took responsibility for making difficult decisions. She felt more comfortable allowing the doctors to manage and control her experience than going through labor and a vaginal birth, and was quite content with Logan's birth.

We are lucky to have the technology that gave Carol her son. Her birth is unique not only in what went right, but also in the opportunities she was denied. There is no doubt that it was all worth it to have Logan arrive safe and sound.

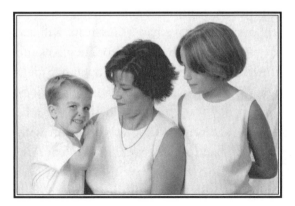

Logan, Carol, and Ashley

CAROL: Ashley, my first child, was due on September 21st. I had her two weeks after my due date, on October 7th. I was scared to do it naturally and I had prepared myself by taking a birth class where we learned about C-sections and by reading the chapter in the book. I went so far past my due date because my body wouldn't do anything for me.

I was huge. To finally induce my labor, I started off with cervical gel, then ended up on Pitocin, which didn't do anything at all. I was one centimeter when I went into the hospital to be induced, and then I went backwards to nothing. My body didn't want to go that way and that was okay. I was scared to do it naturally and I had prepared myself. After inducing me overnight for fourteen hours, we did an ultrasound. It looked like it was going to be a ten-pound baby, so we did the C-section. She was ten pounds, fifteen ounces.

Fear can actually cause the cervix to close, even after dilating. Humans are like any mammal that must have a safe place to give birth; fear releases stress hormones that actually block the birth process. Carol's fear of childbirth was stronger than her body's ability to initiate labor.

Ashley was four when I got pregnant with Logan. Her temperament had postponed a sibling for years. She was a very active, headstrong busybody like her Mom, and I knew that I couldn't take on that much at once. She calmed down and life was a little easier after she turned two years old.

We definitely planned Logan. We originally planned to have our kids a year and a half apart. I liked the close bond that Ron and his sister have, which I do not have with my brothers and sisters. But it took us a year to get pregnant. At first, I didn't really stress over it because I knew what I was getting myself into the second time around,

But something was questionable to me. I went to see my family doctor and had my annual exam and a Pap test. Then she referred me to Dr. P, a gynecology specialist, to discuss the question of why I wasn't getting pregnant. I went into his office about the infertility right about the same time my Pap results came back. My family doctor had called and told him the results, and Dr. P was the one who told me.

I don't remember his exact words. It was a bad result—questionable cancer. He had said the "C word": cancer. It was hard because I was in his office for a whole other reason. All of the sudden, pregnancy was on the back burner. I'd have to wait probably another six months, get results, get healed, and then start talking about pregnancy again. He wanted to do the biopsy right then and there to get things moving pretty fast. But I couldn't do it that quickly. I needed to prepare myself mentally for the biopsy. I had had a hard enough time having a Pap smear done.

I decided to squeeze the biopsy appointment in before my period, which was due in three or four days. If not, it meant having to wait for at least another week. So we did it two days later.

It wasn't as bad as I thought it was going to be. He even made a joke when we were doing it, "You're not pregnant are you?" and I said, "That's why I'm coming to you, because I'm not getting pregnant!" Unusually, I bled a lot after the biopsy and he had to apply pressure for a good twenty minutes before it would stop. We didn't know why.

As long as cervical cancer has not spread to surrounding organs, as in carcinoma in situ, it is easily treated by removing the cancerous cells on the cervix. That is why women must get regular Pap tests, to catch these cells before they spread. But it was the combination of a new pregnancy along with the need for a procedure that made this a tricky situation.

I never did start my period. I truthfully was not surprised. I thought it was the stress of worrying about cancer, finding out my aunt had died of cervical cancer, and the fact that my sister had cervical and uterine cancer when she found out she was eight weeks pregnant. I was pretty stressed and scared. My aunt had been forty and my sister even younger. I was almost twenty-nine.

I got the biopsy results and the term they used was "carcinoma in situ." It wasn't invasive. So we scheduled laser surgery to have it cut away.

I still hadn't started my period, and I was scheduled to see my family doctor on a Friday. I had been baking the night before, and the smell of crescent rolls made me sick. I went in the next day to see my doctor, and I really expected the test to be negative. I was eight days late. Usually if I'm a day late and I'm trying to get pregnant, I'm going in the very next day because I can't wait for anything! But I really didn't think I was pregnant. And then it was positive. I remember it as if it were yesterday. Honestly. Because I cried. I wasn't even happy being pregnant. I was scared being pregnant. Not happy at all.

I had cancer of the cervix and I was supposed to have the surgery to have it cut away. So I thought I was going to be faced with a very tough decision that my sister had been faced with: aborting a baby. And this baby was very, very wanted for a long time.

I was really afraid, excited, scared, and sad—I had every basic emotion. I made the decision, "I'm going to have this baby." I called the hospital, cancelled the surgery, called Dr. P's office and told them I wasn't having it and the reason why. He was on a two-week vacation so he had no idea. Before he got back, I went on the Internet to find any kind of information about cancer and pregnancy, and I saw too often that the survival rate was low. It turns into invasive cancer.

I thought to myself, "That's not fair for Ron if I die in five years because it has spread like wildfire." I couldn't do that to him. I was so stubborn; I was *going* to have this baby. I talked it over with Ron even before Dr. P called me back. I decided I would have the surgery and if I lost the baby, I lost the baby, but I wasn't going to abort. Nothing is ever easy, and nothing is ever simple.

Dr. P also said that I should have the surgery, so I scheduled it again. We did it in the hospital because of the risk involved with bleeding. I was eight weeks pregnant when we did a laser excision of my cervix.

It wasn't bad at all. Most patients get a little local anesthetic, but he wanted me to be comfortable and really reduce the risk of blood loss, so he gave me a spinal. I didn't feel a thing, not then and not afterwards. I bled, but not a lot. The pathology came back saying he had gotten all of it.

I was pretty guarded the first week. He said that it was going to be a really rough time—real iffy. But he said that he couldn't even find any research on doing the procedure and being pregnant so he couldn't say for sure. There was all kinds of information about having cancer during pregnancy, but nothing about doing the surgery during pregnancy. So I was on bed rest, pretty much flat on my back, for a week.

I started mentally preparing myself and disconnecting myself from the pregnancy—not to the point that I wasn't going to bond but to the point that if I lost it I was going to be okay. I had had a previous miscarriage long before Ashley was born, so I knew how it felt. That miscarriage was at sixteen weeks and was pretty devastating. So I told myself that if God wanted me to have this baby, the baby would make it.

My family doctor told me not to lift anything heavier than a full gallon of milk, about two and a half pounds, until told otherwise. Ron brought laundry to me from the dryer and I sat on the couch and folded it. As far as housework, I was not to do anything until I was told that I was okay. I was checked every single day for a few days after the surgery and then every week until it was healed. Then I had to get up into the stirrups every two weeks for a long time when I went to Dr. P. He checked internally, put in a speculum and made sure the cervix was closed.

I was probably between three and three and a half months pregnant when the ordinary risks in the first trimester plus this extra-high risk were no longer in play. I was able to resume a lot of activity, but I was still going in every two weeks to be checked. I didn't obsess. I didn't get paranoid. I didn't think of it all the time because that was going to be worse for me and for the baby. If I did, I would worry. I was getting nervous if I had too much time on my hands to think about it. I wasn't going to be miserable for my whole pregnancy. I didn't do anything really crazy, but I led a normal life. I was careful about some things.

I felt great in my fifth month. Despite all the things I could have problems with, being high risk, I felt much better being pregnant the second time around. I had more energy than I did when I was pregnant before. I was able to do a lot of things. In my fifth month, I did a major spring cleaning in my house.

Dr. P probably didn't know, but I felt like I was doing great. No complications so far. At about six months, he stopped having me come every two weeks, and I thought it was going to be okay. I felt extremely good knowing the baby could now survive outside of my body. Granted it's not the best thing, but it could survive. I knew, "Okay now I can do what I want."

Things stayed exactly the same. Then, around Super Bowl Sunday, when I was six months pregnant, I started having lots of contractions. I sat down and timed them, and they were about five minutes apart. I let it go on for a while and then I called. They had me go into the hospital, and they put the monitor on. I was having quite a few contractions, so they gave me a shot of terbutaline. It made me all jittery, flushed, and warm, but the contractions stopped. Then they sent me home to rest and "take it easy" but the contractions never came back and I was able to get right back up and start doing things. I probably rested for about three or four days and that was enough for me.

I felt good. I wasn't getting as big as I did with Ashley; I don't know why. We knew we were having a boy because I had several ultrasounds. I think that really helped, too. I wanted to plan because I knew that towards the end of my pregnancy I could be flat on my back to keep this baby inside of me in case my cervix did open up. We had the room set up by the time I was five months pregnant. I had the basics for a baby, just in case I couldn't shop later. We named him Logan Christopher before he came out of my stomach. And I think that helped me cope.

Logan never did make up his mind on his position. Every time we checked him he would either be head up or head down or transverse. In the end, when it got close to my due date of May 13th, he was head up. He was backwards. He wasn't moving any more and he wasn't giving us the option for a VBAC (vaginal birth after a C-section).

Dr. P didn't even try to turn him around because of all the other complications and because I had had a previous C-section. He recommended a C-section. It was a week or two ahead of my due date, and I didn't want to continue being pregnant. I was a lot more sore in my pelvic region the second time around, even though I felt good in a lot of other ways. I was ready. I wanted to have him on the first of May but that was too far away from my due date. Dr. P wanted him on the fifth of May. I said, "That just gives my son an extra reason to party on Cinco de Mayo, so we're not going to do that either!" So we came up with a good one: May 4th.

I wasn't scared of another C-section. I had my family doctor, Dr. P, and the same anesthesiologist. It was going to be the same thing all over again. The experience with Ashley's C-section was actually a fun thing. I guess

The days after a C-section are not as easy as those that follow a vaginal birth. Once we take over for Mother Nature, we have to manage complications with the medical model, and this can affect both mother and baby during the first few days after a birth.

that it's probably hard for someone to imagine that being fun, but when you're sharing jokes and people are laughing and it's a celebration, it's fun, for a surgery.

The pain wasn't that bad after that first birth, but when my blood pressure went up to 170/110, I had to go on IV medicine. The magnesium in it made me hallucinate. I had a catheter in and the nurse had to take care of Ashley for several days. I was in the hospital for six days. Plus, I needed anti-nausea medicine right after the birth and it knocked me out. I don't even remember seeing her until five hours later. Thank God for the pictures.

But I wasn't going to have that happen again. I wasn't going to take any anti-nausea medicine, even if it killed me. I was going to be awake, alert, and ready to see my baby. So, only for those reasons was I a little scared of the second C-section; but Dr. P pretty much reassured me that the second one was cushy and the chances of the blood-pressure problem happening again were pretty slim. So I had a really strong mindset about how things were going to go. That helped.

Logan was seven pounds, nine and a half ounces.

I had a good recovery with Logan, I was awake and able to see him and nurse him. As it turns out, I did get nauseated when I sat up to see him. I pretty much threw up for about four hours. But I still didn't take any medication until I was ready to go to bed. I had a spinal for both C-sections. The first time I got severe headaches from it. The second time they assured me that it wouldn't happen because the needles were smaller. And I didn't get any headaches. My blood pressure did get a little borderline but I wrote it off. I kept a very strong mindset that I wasn't going to be in bed for six days. I was up in ten hours, without the catheter, walking the hallways. I made sure I walked and walked and walked so I would get better fast. I was not going to go through the same thing again.

About two months after Ashley was born, I got depressed. It was a subtle thing; I can see it more clearly looking back on it. I couldn't make it through the day. You know, at the beginning you go through the normal "boo hoos," but it was extreme with her. It was fatigue and frustration. I couldn't get her to nurse right, to latch on, my tummy was sore, and I couldn't put her on my tummy. Then when the newness of the baby wore off, it was just work. I was mentally wiped out at the end of the day, drinking some wine just to be able to cope. I didn't do anything medication wise. I didn't see my family doctor about it. It wasn't that bad, but I just wasn't happy.

It was a lot different with Logan. It was a lot harder. Logan did nothing but cry the first two days. I called my family doctor at four in the morning saying, "This kid has not slept. He's done nothing but cry." I thought there was something wrong with him. Right after that I remember crying, and Ron saying, "What's wrong with you?" and I'd say, "I'm okay, I just can't stop. I feel okay. I just can't stop crying, so let me cry." So I cried for probably an hour straight and felt good afterwards. I did go through a hormonal shift afterwards with sweats and things like that but it didn't bother me emotionally. I just knew it was a natural process. It lasted a couple of months and it ended subtly, like it started.

In theory I'd love to have more children. I was ready to have a third one right away. If I could just have a baby and nurse and have people put food underneath my nose, I would do it a lot. I love that beginning, just having them, meeting them for the first time, and nursing them for the first time. I loved the bonding, the emotional part, the high. I could do that over and over and over. I could skip the pregnancy, but I love having the baby, even if it's by C-section. I never felt guilty about not doing it the other way. I was okay with that.

Logan's whole birth story had a good, happy ending. My life doesn't always give that to me, but I really felt like he was a miracle when he got here.

Fear of birthing naturally was a significant factor in Carol's choice to have a Cesarean section with her first pregnancy. Cervical cancer created even more fear during her second pregnancy. Once medical technology takes over, it is difficult to back off and allow Mother Nature to lead the way. In Carol's case, Mother Nature was forcing us to interfere, both because of the cancer and the breech positioning.

So much fear leading to lost opportunities is extremely sad, so it was not surprising that Carol dealt with depression after her births. More than once I have seen fear before a birth lead to depression afterwards. The two emotions are closely connected. My wish for Carol, if I could have changed something, would be for her to have had less to fear and the opportunity to experience more power and joy during her births.

Pregnancy and birth can teach us lessons about life and ourselves— lessons that prepare us for parenting. We learn to face uncertainty and loss of control. Sometimes we are fearful but find that we can be courageous in the face of our fear. Carol knew her fear, and in giving the control to her doctors, she found the support she needed to be brave. Her two wonderful children continue to provide her ample opportunity to experience abundant joy.

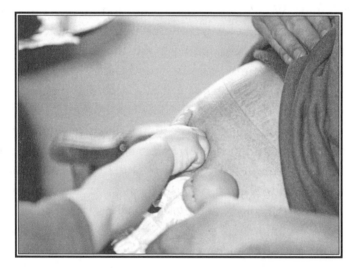

FOR PHYSICIANS—HOW TO BE AN
INTEGRATIVE CHILDBIRTH PROVIDER

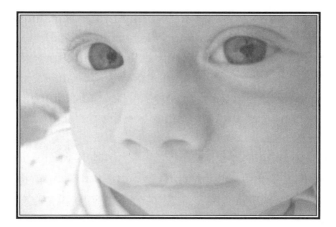

Just as a woman in labor may believe that she is unable to give birth without medical intervention, so too may physicians believe they are unable to assist the birthing process without technology. Many physicians have never seen a natural childbirth, having trained in tertiary-care facilities that medically manage every birth with fetal monitors, Pitocin, and strict hospital protocols. But allowing women the opportunity to experience a natural childbirth is a gift that will help her for years to come. Guiding a child to maturity takes patience, perseverance, courage, the ability to give up control, a sense of humor, great respect for partners, and a lot of faith. If you support your patients through a natural birth, you also allow them to experience their first valuable lessons in parenting.

Without faith in the natural birthing process, it is almost impossible to support integrative childbirth. *I encourage all physicians who assist women in having babies to get as much experience as they can with natural birth.* Observe and learn from midwives, attend births at birth centers, and learn all you can about births that are successful without the use of any medications or interventions. Build a trust in the human body that you can share with your patients. Keep your skills sharp, just in case you need them, but keep the medical model in the background.

The midwifery model of care was defined in an earlier chapter, but because of its importance it bears repeating here. As stated by the Midwifery Task Force in 1996, "The *midwifery model of care* is based on the assumption that pregnancy and birth are normal life events. This model of care includes monitoring the physical, psychological, and social wellbeing of the mother throughout the childbearing cycle; providing the mother with individualized education, counseling, and prenatal care, continuous hands-on assistance during labor and delivery, and postpartum support; minimizing technological interventions; and identifying and referring women who require obstetrical attention. The application of this woman-centered model has been proven to reduce the incidence of birth injury, trauma, and cesarean section."

The medical model of maternity care considers pregnancy and labor unstable physical conditions. Medical intervention is an integral part of every birth, and birth is virtually never considered a completely safe process. The ever present possibility of legal action triggered by alleged mismanagement affects medical decisions. Women's labors and deliveries are compared to statistical expectations, and any deviation from these expectations is a cause for concern. Birth is seen as a physical process, not a spiritual or emotional one, so managing it with aggressive technology is considered appropriate medical care. Because the pains of childbirth are considered unnecessarily grueling, the use of pain medication and anesthesia are the norm.

We should base our initial care plan on the midwifery model. If we combine clear patient communication with a sound knowledge of normal childbirth and use technology only when necessary to serve the needs of laboring mothers, we have a true integration: the best of both worlds.

If you are a physician, you will quickly place yourself somewhere on the continuum between the two purest extremes. You might already see yourself as providing integrative care, having found it more personally satisfying and knowing it to be good medicine. You may have seen many normal and natural births and are comfortable with individualized care. Maybe you want to have a style that is more like a midwife's but feel forced to practice in a world of medicine that demands the aggressive use of technology. Maybe you value what technology has to offer, feeling comfortable with the sense of control the medical model offers. Finding your place along this continuum and matching your style to your individual patient's needs is the goal of a physician practicing integrative childbirth.

Research has shown that the integrative childbirth model increases patient safety and decreases the physician's risk of liability by focusing on the individual and her family.[2,3,4,5] When the midwifery model of care is applied, between eighty-five and ninety-five percent of healthy women safely give birth without surgery or other hospital-based interventions.[6] Medical interventions come into play as part of sensible pregnancy monitoring and during labor and delivery. Intervention is inappropriate unless it is truly necessary, and it may actually be harmful when it is used purely for patient or physician convenience, or for profit.

Integrative childbirth requires that the provider spend enough time with each patient to build a relationship. If you do not want a personal relationship with your patients, stop reading this chapter right now— you probably are not really interested in providing this type of care. But before you give up the idea as ludicrous or impossible, consider the very real benefits of this personal relationship: less likelihood of litigation and a high likelihood that you will gain immense satisfaction from your practice. Your relationships with your patients may remind you of your reasons for choosing medicine as a career in the first place.

---

2. Eastaugh SR. Reducing litigation costs through better patient communication. *Physician Exec.* May-Jun 2004;30(3):36-38.

3. Forster HP, Schwartz J, DeRenzo E. Reducing legal risk by practicing patient-centered medicine. *Arch Intern Med.* Jun 10 2002;162(11):1217-1219.

4. Saxton JW. How to increase economic returns and reduce liability exposure: Part 1—Patient satisfaction as an economic tool. *J Med Pract Manage.* Nov-Dec 2001;17(3):142-144.

5. Terry K. Telling patients more will save you time. *Med Econ.* Jul 25 1994;71(14):40, 43, 46 passim.

6. *BMJ* 2005;330:1416 (18 June), doi:10.1136/bmj.330.7505.1416.

PRACTICE-MANAGEMENT FOR INTEGRATIVE CHILDBIRTH CARE

The following five steps will allow a physician to practice integrative childbirth:

1. Perform intake interviews and initial physical exams personally. The half-hour this takes saves hours of time later.

2. Do all your own prenatal exams. You can limit them to ten or fifteen minutes each if you make use of that time wisely. Regular visits provide enough time to establish communication and trust.

3. If you share a call schedule with others, share obstetrics call with providers who practice this style of childbirth.

4. Work in a hospital that knows your style of practice (or is willing to learn it), knows that integrative childbirth is good medicine, and honors your judicious use of protocols. Develop communication and trust with the hospital staff and nurses—they are a valuable extension of you and your care.

5. Make sure your patients' needs and expectations match your own style of care. If not, either change your style to fit that particular patient or recommend that they transfer their care to another provider.

These practice-management elements are feasible, even in a busy family practice or obstetric clinic. Obstetrics is a high-risk part of a physician's practice. It is a well known and well supported fact that physician-patient communication problems are behind most malpractice claims. Adjusting your schedule to accommodate integrative childbirth will actually decrease your malpractice risk and increase your personal satisfaction. This is a win–win situation!

ESSENTIAL ELEMENTS OF STYLE

But of course, there is more to integrative care than practice management. Now consider the four key style elements involved in practicing integrative prenatal care and childbirth. I call them the Four Cs for Physicians: Communication, Continuity, Confidence, and Control of Protocols.

COMMUNICATION

Clear communication at each prenatal visit builds realistic expectations and an essential foundation for difficult decisions that may be needed during the intensity of a birth.

Many doctors have their nurses obtain intake information about each newly pregnant woman. You may have the patient fill out information forms and then review this information later, when the patients are gone and you have the opportunity to go over charts. There are usually several pages of background information to gather, and it takes time to record all this data. But in integrative childbirth, I cannot overstate the importance of getting this information yourself. This is the first step to integrative childbirth.

The half-hour it takes to gather this information personally is well worth the payoff in creating the relationship you'll need seven months later. You want your patients to trust you and to learn how to openly communicate with you; you want a functional working relationship with the family when this woman goes into labor. During this visit, you may openly discuss family support, possible religious limitations, and past history that may affect the pregnancy. You will get a sense of how the couple works together, how they solve problems together, and what their personalities bring to the situation.

This initial meeting gives you an opportunity to ask the couple to think about family and community support in case the pregnancy develops complications. Some high-risk situations require bed rest, and you don't want a couple to be completely unprepared to handle a difficult pregnancy. In this way you also get an idea of how large their community is and how others may be able to help them during the pregnancy. There may be a well-meaning relative who would love to help out but whose visit would be more stressful than helpful, and discussing such possibilities is a good start in forming an alliance with the family. In my practice, we laugh about these thoughts of trouble, and I always say it is like carrying an umbrella to make sure it doesn't rain. But there are times when that part of our initial conversation makes difficult decisions easier, later in the pregnancy.

During this initial visit, you should also explain your style of care to the mother-to-be and her partner. If they expect something different than what you have to offer, they should find a more suitable provider sooner rather than later. My style has always been hands-on watchfulness: letting Mother Nature have her way, watching with vigilance for any signs of problems, and addressing problems as the need arises. I make it clear that I will do nothing unless there is an obvious need. I order all the necessary lab tests, order sonograms only if indicated, and explain the "why" of everything I recommend.

I explain all reasonable care options and allow them to choose what is right for them. I also explain that I am a medical doctor and therefore have a responsibility to provide a certain standard of care. Certain tests, such as screening for diabetes, are not negotiable because in my opinion, they are necessary for safe care. If they sincerely want either a more or a less aggressive approach to their pregnancy or labor, I will refer them to another provider. Above all, I want them to trust the provider they choose to work with.

After the first visit, you should personally see each woman for a brief but focused fifteen-minute visit once a month. It is important for the provider to perform these prenatal visits personally rather than expecting others to do the job. Even ten minutes of a physician's undivided attention can feel like a half-hour of communication to the patient and her family. Fifteen minutes is plenty of time to check her belly, measure it, listen to the heartbeat, and discuss her concerns about the pregnancy.

Ask that she bring in a list of questions when she comes to see you; this makes each visit more efficient. Have your own list of items ready to discuss at each stage of pregnancy: necessary screening tests, sonograms, and plans for the delivery. Being able to address most of her concerns before she gets a chance to ask is a sign that you are building the relationship you need, but always ask if there is anything she or her partner want to talk about that you have not already covered. Make direct eye contact, sit down when appropriate, and allow the patient to talk uninterrupted for longer than a minute or two at a time.

If communication is clear, by the ninth month you will probably have answered every question the family can think of. You will have created a relationship that allows you to work well with this family during the labor and delivery. And should you find an inability to communicate or a serious incompatibility, you will have figured this out long before you go in to deliver their baby.

CONTINUITY

Continuity of care is one of the main reasons patients choose midwives rather than physicians to deliver their babies. Doing your own prenatal exams provides prenatal continuity, but promising to be the one to deliver the baby is difficult for many physicians. Keeping up with deliveries that happen in the middle of a busy clinic day or in the middle of the night is stressful and demanding, and being on call for all deliveries all the time is often impossible. Many doctors are overloaded with call schedules and with full clinic schedules, so it is becoming increasingly rare for patients to have the provider who sees her at her prenatal visits be there when she goes into labor. Groups of physicians share call, and no one knows who will deliver a baby until the mother is in labor.

However, with integrative childbirth, it is essential for the mother to know and trust the person who is delivering her baby. Ideally, the physician who has provided all the prenatal care will do the delivery, but continuity can still be accomplished by having continuity of style. Your call partners need to offer the same type of delivery experience that you yourself provide: full communication, no interventions unless necessary, and a reliance on established trust when intervention is needed. Introduce your patients to the other providers in the call group who have similar styles of practice. During the last month of pregnancy, the prenatal visits are usually scheduled weekly. Some of these visits can be scheduled with your call partners so that they are not strangers should they be the ones present at the time of delivery.

CONFIDENCE AND TRUST

The pregnant woman must trust her provider with her life, and with the life of her baby. She must have confidence that you will keep the agreements you made during the months of prenatal care. The woman seeking integrative childbirth wants to trust her provider to care for her emotional well-being in addition to her physical needs. She expects to be told the truth, she expects full communication, and she should not have to defend herself while she is in labor.

Similarly, your patients must trust you enough to be honest and communicative with you throughout the pregnancy. They need to know they can speak freely and be heard. During the birth, with all the added stressors of nervous family members, the busy hospital staff, and the realities of labor, this trust will be the cornerstone of an integrative childbirth.

Trust is built over time and will follow naturally if you encourage honest and open communication. It is important for the family to have confidence in you. If there is time and opportunity, everything you do during labor will be explained and agreed upon prior to acting—but in the case of a sudden emergency, you must have the family's permission to act quickly and without negotiation. If either you or your patient admits to a serious lack of confidence, this should be addressed and a change in providers should be considered long before the membranes rupture.

CONTROL OF PROTOCOLS

There is one more quality that is essential in an integrative-childbirth health care provider—the knowledge that protocols are not people. Prenatal management is full of protocols. Physicians spend hours in committees creating extensive lists of recommended rules for managing all kinds of medical problems associated with pregnancy, labor, and delivery. The recommendations are based on experience, statistical risk factors, and current studies of pregnant women. Some of these protocols make sense and are not only valid, but essential, for quality care; others are for special situations that affect a minority of women. But individual women may not want to be managed by protocols that are not dictated by their individual needs or preferences.

The most common way a laboring woman loses power is by being given homogenous care based on hospital protocols. The continuous use of monitors, loss of mobility, rigid expectations of a time line for labor, and use of medications—all of these may not be necessary for the laboring woman. The physician that promises to consider the individual and her unique labor needs will gain an immense amount of trust from her patient.

As a provider offering integrative childbirth, you should be the patient's advocate in the hospital. If the mother wants minimal intervention, use only those procedures that are necessary to her unique situation. Explain the hospital's protocols to her ahead of time so that she can work with the staff when she gets to the hospital; it is important for the staff to feel that they have enough freedom to provide a safe birth. Communicating about these expectations prior to the birth day is important. If trust is established, explaining the need for some protocols should be simple, and they should be easily accepted.

The fear of protocols and resulting loss of power leads people to create their own birth plan—their own set of personal protocols for this birth. Birth plans are important documents and should be taken seriously. Sometime in the last month of prenatal care, you and the family should review their written birth plan, discuss any anticipated problems, and agree on realistic and mutual expectations. Take their plan seriously, agree to work with them to edit it as necessary, and clearly explain any aspects that may cause problems.

For example, many women say they do not want to be strapped to a fetal monitor while they are in labor, and this may be clearly stated in their birth plans. I happen to agree that it is not good for a normal laboring woman to be immobilized by technology. On the other hand, I do want the reassurance of a good fetal heart rate periodically. I recommend an initial fifteen-minute monitor check (for everyone's reassurance on admission), then brief periodic (hourly) checks on the baby's heartbeat as long as things are going well.

I have never had a mother refuse periodic checks on her baby's well-being. If I honor her need to labor freely and she honors our need to know that her baby appears well, we arrive at a plan that ensures that everyone's needs are met. Hospital protocols are followed, the staff is reassured, and the laboring mother keeps her mobility.

However, we have a saying in my practice: "Burn the birth plan!" My patients were the ones who coined this phrase when they realized during their labors that Mother Nature had her own ideas. They knew a change of plans was always a possibility, and I'd be sure to include this idea in our discussions of birth plans. Rigid attachment to any birth scenario is not helpful to either the laboring mother or her caregivers, and the initial discussion of birth plans is the perfect time to talk about going with the flow of a natural birth.

Fostering communication, continuity, confidence, and control of protocols are all part of practicing exceptionally good medicine, along with a good dose of common sense. Integrative childbirth practices do take time and dedication. So why dedicate your time and energy to this style of obstetrics? The answer lies in who you are, the kind of care you want to provide, and the reasons you decided to deliver babies in the first place.

If you have faith in the birthing process and faith in your ability to help that process when needed, you are a good candidate for providing integrative childbirth. If you are open to creating a close personal relationship with your patients that will support them during a delivery, no matter what surprises Mother Nature has in store, integrative childbirth is a good choice. It is the safest and sanest way to practice the art of medicine—full of respect for the patient and the miracle we are honored to attend.

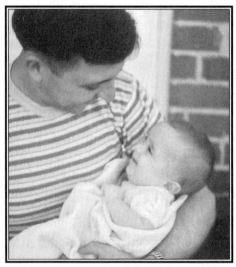

The author and her father

ACKNOWLEDGEMENTS

PHOTO CREDITS

Denise Axtell: *page 168*

Heather Bussing: *page 100*

Terri Cookston: *pages 66, 73, 75, 107, 108, 109, 110, 142, 143, 144, 166, 180, 187, 190*

M. Chrissy Gardella-Hester: *page 173 and cover photo*

Donna Heald: *page 88*

David Hester: *page 142 (portrait)*

Elke Hodges: *pages 154 and 158*

Barbara Kerr: *page 208*

Stacey Kerr MD: *pages 15, 31, 40, 78, 86, 98, 111, 122, 123, 125, 146, 199*

Dylan Moore: *page 17*

Jean Porter: *pages 29 and 42*

Laura Viramontes: *page 136*

Additional acknowledgement to Elizabeth Koebsell, for tireless transcribing, and to Dorothy Wall, for her endless edits and encouragement—thank you!

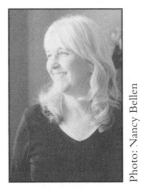

Photo: Nancy Bellen

ABOUT THE AUTHOR

Stacey Marie Kerr, MD, is a family physician who has provided family-centered childbirth experiences for her patients for more than fifteen years.

During the 1970s and early '80s, Dr. Kerr lived on The Farm, an intentional spiritual community in Summertown, Tennessee, known for its midwifery skills. While there, she collected statistics for Ina May Gaskin's groundbreaking book, *Spiritual Midwifery*.

In 1989, at the age of thirty-nine, Dr. Kerr graduated with an MD from the University of California, Davis, Medical School. She completed her residency and earned her Board Certification in Family Medicine in 1992, probably the first grandmother to graduate from the Santa Rosa UCSF residency program. Dr. Kerr has two children, both natural childbirths. Her first was born at a birthing center in central Missouri and the second was born at home on The Farm.

Dr. Kerr has been published extensively in medical journals, including *JAMA*, *California Family Physician*, and *Sonoma Medicine*. She writes a monthly health column for the *Santa Rosa Press Democrat*. She served for two years as state chair of the Public Outreach Committee for the California Academy of Family Physicians, and two years as chair of the credentialing committee at her local hospital, which allowed her to credential midwives for hospital staff privileges. She lives in Santa Rosa, California, and her website is www.homebirthinthehospital.com.